FOOD AND BEVERAGE CONSUMPTION AND HEALTH SERIES

FRUIT AND VEGETABLE CONSUMPTION AND HEALTH

FOOD AND BEVERAGE CONSUMPTION AND HEALTH SERIES

Handbook of Green Tea and Health Research
Helen McKinley and Mark Jamieson (Editors)
2009. ISBN: 978-1-60741-045-4

Handbook of Green Tea and Health Research (E-Book)
Helen McKinley and Mark Jamieson (Editors)
2009. ISBN: 978-1-60876-202-6

Marketing Food to Children and Adolescents
Nicoletta A. Wilks
2009. ISBN: 978-1-60692-913-1

Food Labelling: The FDA's Role in the Selection of Healthy Foods
Ethan C. Lefevre (Editor)
2009. ISBN: 78-1-60692-898-1

Fish Consumption and Health
George P. Gagne and Richard H. Medrano (Editors)
2009. ISBN: 978-1-60741-151-2

Alcoholic Beverage Consumption and Health
Adam Mazzei and Agostina D'Arco (Editors)
2009. ISBN: 978-1-60741-160-4

Milk Consumption and Health
Ebbe Lange and Felix Vogel (Editors)
2009. ISBN: 978-1-60741-459-9

Red Wine and Health
Paul O'Byrne (Editor)
2009. ISBN: 978-1-60692-718-2

Red Wine and Health (E-Book)
Paul O'Byrne (Editor)
2009. ISBN: 978-1-60741-284-7

Fruit Juices: Properties, Consumption and Nutrition
Pauline G. Scardina (Editors)
2009. ISBN: 978-1-60741-505-3

Fruit and Vegetable Consumption and Health
Anton Papareschi and Harvey Eppolito (Editors)
2009. ISBN: 978-1-60741-596-1

FOOD AND BEVERAGE CONSUMPTION AND HEALTH SERIES

FRUIT AND VEGETABLE CONSUMPTION AND HEALTH

ANTON PAPARESCHI
AND
HARVEY EPPOLITO
EDITORS

Nova Science Publishers, Inc.
New York

For permission to use material from this book please contact us:
Telephone 631-231-7269; Fax 631-231-8175
Web Site: http://www.novapublishers.com

Library of Congress Cataloging-in-Publication Data

Fruit and vegetable consumption and health / [edited by] Anton Papareschi and Harvey Eppolito.
p. cm.
Includes index.
ISBN 978-1-60741-596-1 (hardcover)
1. Fruit in human nutrition. 2. Vegetables in human nutrition. I. Papareschi, Anton. II. Eppolito, Harvey.
QP144.F78F77 2009
613.2--dc22

2009025480

Published by Nova Science Publishers, Inc. ✦ New York

Contents

Preface

Fruit and vegetables are important components of a healthy diet, and their sufficient daily consumption could help prevent major diseases, such as cardiovascular diseases and certain cancers. Overall, it is estimated that up to 2.7 million lives could potentially be saved each year if fruit and vegetable consumption were sufficiently increased. A recently published World Health Organization (WHO) report recommends as a population-wide intake goal the consumption of a minimum of 400g of fruit and vegetables per day (excluding potatoes and other starchy tubers) for the prevention of chronic diseases such as heart disease, cancer, diabetes and obesity, as well as for the prevention and alleviation of several micronutrient deficiencies, especially in less developed countries. The WHO Global Strategy on Diet, Physical Activity and Health emphasizes the increase of fruit and vegetables consumption as one of the dietary recommendations to be considered when preparing national policies and dietary guidelines for populations and individuals. This new book gathers the latest research from around the globe in this field of study.

Chapter I - Fruit and greens are traditional components of the Brazilian diet and their uneventful consumption has been stimulated in several countries, as the consumers perceive them as healthy, tasteful, convenient and fresh foods. They are vitamin sources, besides having compounds with antioxidant action, as lycopen, lutein and alpha-carotene that, at cellular level, hinder the accumulation of free radicals, minimizing the cancer occurrence (Fahrasmane et al., 2007). Williamson (1996) verified that an increase of consumption of leaf vegetables (cauliflower, broccoli) was related to a reduction of risk of developing cancer in the intestine and in the thyroid. Musgrove (2008) reports that the medium number of present portions of vegetables and fruit in England was 3.1 and an increase in the number of children ingesting five or more portions was observed (Musgrove, 2008). Another study performed in the United States reports that 55% of people believe that compounds naturally present in these foods may help to prevent diseases, being reported the consumers' preference for their ingestion (Childs and Poryzees, 1998). Consequently, the food industry, researches and consumers have been showing great interest in the antioxidant power of phlavonoids, anthocyanins and other present phytochemical compounds which can have protecting effect against cancer and cardiovascular diseases (Ness and Powles, 1997).

Chapter II - Toxic elements e.g., arsenic (As), cadmium (Cd), chromium (Cr), copper (Cu), lead (Pb), and zinc (Zn) are the chief environmental pollutants which can cause deleterious health effects in humans. Inhalation and consumption of metal-contaminated food are the major pathways of metal entrance into human body. Cultivation of crop plants in the metal-contaminated soils induces the bioaccumulation of toxic elements in the food chain. Among different food items, vegetables have major contribution in the daily diet, and the heavy metal contamination of vegetables poses a threat to human health with the prevalence of skin and gastrointerestinal cancer.

The uptake and bioaccumulation of toxic elements in vegetables are influenced by a number of factors such as atmospheric deposition, metal concentrations in soil, soil characteristics, and duration of cultivation. Cultivation areas near highways are exposed to atmospheric pollution in the form of metal containing aerosols which can be deposited on leaves of vegetables and then absorbed. The magnitude of heavy metal deposition on vegetable surfaces varied with morpho-physiological nature of the vegetables. Post-harvest activities, such as transportation, marketing, cooking, etc., may also influence the deposition of toxic elements in vegetables. Incorporation of toxic elements during transportation and marketing of vegetable can be occurred due to the use of contaminated water. Higher heavy metal content in vegetables from urban area then those from rural areas may be due to the contribution of urban activities which elevates heavy metal loads in atmospheric deposition and consequently in the edible part of the vegetables. Cooking has definite influence to the content of toxic elements in cooked items if the heavy metal concentrations in the cooking water are high.

Vegetable consumption varies with age group, food habit, as well as vegetable availability. For example the mean daily vegetable consumption among the European people is 153 g (ranged between 109-241 g) while it is around 250g among the South Asian people. Vegetables occupy a substantial proportion of the daily diet for the South-East Asian people, especially the Japanese, Korean and Chinese people. Thus, whatever the metal contents in vegetables are, their intake in human is, off course, dependent on the total vegetable consumption. In this review, the contribution of vegetables in dietary intake of toxic elements has been discussed from a common platform.

Chapter III - *Background:* Epidemiological evidence suggests that populations with high vegetable and fruit (VF) consumption (>5 portions/day) have a lower risk of developing childhood obesity, cancer, and cardiovascular diseases. In Mexico there is a dearth of information that identifies the determinants of VF intake in children. The aim of the present study was to assess the number of portions consumed by and the determinants of VF intake among children and their parents in a sample of Mexico City's public schools.

Methods: The authors administered two previously tested and validated questionnaires for children and their parents (Cronbach's *alpha* 0.84 and 0.74) respectively. The authors also administered a validated two-day dietary recall used to assess VF intake and its correlates among 327 children and a group of 142 parents.

Results: Among study participant, children consumed approximately one portion of VF per day. Girls consumed more VF than boys ($p<0.01$). Parents consumed four daily portions. Environmental factors that influenced a higher consumption of VF among children include: mothers being in charge of cooking the meals at home ($p<0.02$) and accessibility to VF (<0.01). Personal variables were self-efficacy ($p<0.05$) and vegetable preference ($p<0.03$). Being a girl (OR 2.2, CI: 1.04-4.7), accessibility to VF (OR 3.38, CI: 1.26-9.0) and total VF consumption among parents (OR 1.37, CI:1.08-1.7) were the determinants of VF consumption in the multivariate analysis. The personal and environmental factors that influenced a higher VF consumption among parents were knowledge ($p<0.05$) and vegetable preference (<0.01). Knowledge (OR 1.63, CI: 1.23-2.17) was the determinant of VF consumption among parents in the multivariate model.

Conclusion: The characteristics that correlate with VF consumption among children attending Mexico City's public school system include, being a girl, accessibility to VF and total VF consumption in parents. VF consumption for parents was correlated with knowledge. These factors should be considered when designing public policies aimed increasing VF consumption among children and their parents.

Chapter IV - Type 2 diabetes and cancer are among the leading causes of death in the United States, and the etiology of both diseases is linked to dietary intake. This chapter includes an overview of the studies that examined the relationships between vegetable consumption, and type 2 diabetes and various cancers. Potential mechanisms of action that might be underlying the associations between vegetable intake and type 2 diabetes or cancer risk have also been discussed. Briefly, several studies point out the probable protective influence of vegetable intake against type 2 diabetes and various cancers. However, not all studies agree on this potential protective effect. Some of this disagreement might be coming from the methodological differences between the studies. It is possible that various nutrients and non-nutrient components in vegetables and other foods might be exerting protective effects cumulatively. Additionally, diets high in vegetables might be replacing less healthful intake patterns or might be related to diabetes and cancer via complex relationships with other lifestyle characteristics and disease risk factors (e.g., obesity). Considering that studies do not indicate any increased risk of type 2 diabetes or cancer with higher non-starchy vegetable consumption, aiming for diets that are higher in non-starchy vegetables seem to be a valuable nutrition and public health strategy.

Chapter V - A recent review of the literature has identified 19 *in-vitro* studies, 4 animal experiments and 3 clinical trials investigating elderberry fruit preparations. The effect profile of elderberry fruit covers antioxidative, antiviral, antiproliferative and possibly anti-inflammatory and antibacterial effects *in vitro*. One animal experiment indicated anti-inflammatory activity. One animal experiment and one clinical trial demonstrated a weak anti-lipidemic effect. The proprietary elderberry fruit product Sambucol^R showed *in vitro* antiviral activity. However, the clinical evidence of antiviral effectiveness is presently only moderate because a confirmatory study is warranted. An increasing number of food supplements prepared from elderberry fruit go along with health claims. Consumers should therefore be fully informed about the benefits, risks and hazards associated with the consumption of elderberry fruit products.

The berries of European elder contain a number of health-promoting compounds. Since anthocyanins are absorbed in low quantities into the systemic circulation, they may be involved in beneficial effects. For transparency reasons, the anthocyanin contents should be declared on food supplements together with the method of analysis. HPLC with diode array and mass spectrometric detection appears to be the most reliable method for the determination of the profile and contents of anthocyanins present in such supplements, whereas spectrophotometric assays provide information only about the sum of compounds absorbing at a given wavelength. Using LC-MS, the authors showed that the anthocyanin content of a proprietary food supplement was negligible. Anthocyanins may be degraded during preparation of the food supplement by the impact of oxygen and heat or react with other constituents present. Selecting *Sambucus* genotypes rich in ascorbic acid and also in flavonols and anthocyanins - harvested at the optimum harvest time - may provide good quality raw materials to be processed into dietary supplements.

The daily doses of elderberry fruit or food products have not yet been systematically evaluated in dose-finding studies with respect to the specific effects. Berries may be toxic, especially for children, and also potentially allergenic. Anthocyanins may have an impact on urinary pH. Further studies are required to rule out that elderberry preparations interfere with renal stone formation. Preclinical safety data are urgently warranted.

Chapter VI - There are no FAO statistics available for loquat production and Consumption, thus, the present data derives from journal publication and from personal communications by experts in producing countries, especially from The 2nd Intern. Symp. on Loquat held at Guangzhou, China on April, 2006.

Loquat is now commercially produced in many countries. There are two big producing regions: eastern to southern Asia and around Mediterranean. The major producing countries are China, Spain, Pakistan, India, Japan and Turkey. China stands out as the main world producer of loquat with a crop area of more than 120,000 ha and annual production of 400,000 tonnes (t). Loquat are now grown in 20 out of 32 provinces, nearly all below 35°N.

The fruiting season now extends from December to Sep. due to incorporation of new regions. Loquat is frequently sold at local markets in China during the fruiting season, mainly from March to June, at a higher price. Fruits can be consumed fresh (more than 80%) or processed (about 5%) and can be used for jam, juice, wine, syrup, or as candied fruits; seeds are rich in starch (20 percent) and have been used to make wine. Loquat is highly nectariforous, with a heavy fragrance and high honey potential.

In Spain, as a consequence of environmental requirements, and for other socio-econnmic reasons, most of the production is located in three areas, namely, Alicante, Andalusia and Palancia. Loquat ripens between March and May, total production is 43,300 t, 36% of them is exported, which account for 85% of international trade of loquat. Loquats are concentrated in Japan's warm districts, including Kyushu and some prefectures of Honshu. Loquat is often the most expensive fruit on the market, reflecting the high cost of production, and is now marketed over a very long season. Although the crop area in Japan declined during and after World War II (only about 10 ,000t per year), protected culture has increased since the 1970s.

Leaves and fruits of loquats traditionally have been considered to have high medicinal value and there is evidence of pharmaceutically active compounds. An alcoholic extract has been shown to exhibit anti-inflammatory and hypoglycemic effects. Compared with some pomes sach as apple, pear and haw, and some tropical and subtropical fruits such as orange, banana, mango, litchi and longan, loquat fruits contained high levels of A vitamins, (537 μgRE), Carotene (322.3μg), Ca, Na and Se (20 Chemical compositions of loquat fruit are presented. A product contained loquat are recommended for chronhi bronchitis, coughs, and lung congestion. Contents are listed as loquat leaves with other herbs.

Besides common loquat (*Eriobotrya japonica* Lindl.), 20 other wild loquat species (such as *E. obovata, E. deflexa,*) in genus *Eriobotrya* are recently examined to have significant amounts of phenolics and flavonoids, and exhibit a strong antioxidant activity.

Chapter VII - The interest of humans for the diet composition and the link of this concern to a healthy status is growing more and more. Thus, the incorporation of some terms/concepts into our background has greatly improved our knowledge on disciplines such as Nutrition, Dietetics, Physiology and even Biochemistry. In this context, the field of antioxidants has gained special attention due to the involvement of these compounds in the defense against some pathologies and in aging processes. Accordingly, the consumption of antioxidants has notably increased in the first world population as complements of the diet. Some of these antioxidants have a vitamin nature, and the intake of multivitamin additives, either as single or incorporated to the food, has become one of the identities of the consumer society. However, the rule of *the more the better* does not fit in nutrition, and this is obvious. An over-consumption of antioxidants may lead to unexpected effects.

Antioxidants refer to those substances which, in little amounts, are able to prevent the oxidation of other molecules thus avoiding dysfunction of these in the metabolism. These oxidations are mainly promoted by reactive oxygen species (ROS), where oxygen free radicals are included. Plants are the source of many antioxidants with important roles in the human physiology. Thus, vitamin C (ascorbic acid, ascorbate), the paradigm of the antioxidants, is present in plant tissues, fungi and some animal species, but primates are unable to synthesize it. This makes humans be plant-dependent beings at this level. Other major plant antioxidants with vitamin nature include □-tocopherol (vitamin E), □-carotene (provitamin A), and flavonoids. The beneficial role of these compounds in the physiology and in pathological situations and their presence in many natural products have addressed the interest towards the research of many plant species which were always included in our diet but, by some unknown reasons, possibly the present life rhythm, were almost forgotten.

In this chapter, the generation of ROS in biological systems and the role of some plant antioxidants in the scavenging of these ROS will be analyzed. A discussion of how these compounds may influence our diet will be also addressed.

Chapter VIII - The Kids Choice Program (Hendy, Williams, and Camise, 2005) was designed as a school-based program to increase children's weight management behaviors while in their everyday environments and while in the company of their peers. The present application of the program targeted two weight management behaviors: eating fruits and vegetables first during the meal (FVFIRST), choosing low-fat and low-sugar healthy drinks (HDRINK). Lunch observations revealed that 82 intervention-group children showed more improvements in both FVFIRST and HDRINK than did 85 control-group children. The Kids Choice Program shows promise for long-term adoption by schools because it is simple in design (children wear nametags, stars are punched into nametags when children choose healthy behaviors, weekly Reward Days let children trade stars for small prizes), because it is relatively low in cost ($2 per child per month of application), and because it is well-accepted by children and their parents.

Chapter IX - Fruits and vegetables are essential components of a healthy diet. However, only limited information is available about the fruit and vegetable intake of older women. This study describes the socio-demographic and health correlates of intake of fruit and vegetables among two large cohorts of Australian women – one group aged 50-55 years and one aged 79-84 years. Almost all women ate some amount of fruit and vegetables each day. In each cohort, around 8-9% of the women ate five or more serves of vegetables each day, and 30% ate four or more serves each day. In the Mid-age cohort, around 60% of the women ate two or more servings of fruit each day, and the corresponding proportion for the older cohort was 70%. Around 7-8% of each cohort could be considered to eat the national recommended intake of two serves of fruit and five serves of vegetables. Eating higher levels of fruit and vegetables was associated with country of birth, education, marital status, and with functional abilities and oral health. Longitudinal analyses describe trends in BMI, health-related quality of life and survival according to women's fruit and vegetable intakes.

Chapter X - The purpose of this study was to provide nutrition educators with a baseline understanding of how preschoolers' current concepts and knowledge of fruits and vegetables relates with their primary care providers (i.e. parents, grandparents, or foster parents) and childcare providers. The exploratory, theory-based, qualitative study design involved interviews with preschoolers (n=24) and their primary care providers (n=22) and childcare providers (n=2). Maps were used to qualitatively compare similarities in responses to questions regarding fruits and vegetables between a preschooler and her primary care provider and childcare provider. The concepts expressed by the preschoolers were shared minimally with their primary care providers and childcare providers. Further work is needed in understanding how to utilize primary care providers and childcare providers and the underlying preschool contextual setting to increase preschoolers' concepts and knowledge of fruits and vegetables.

In: Fruit and Vegetable Consumption and Health
Editors: Anton Papareschi and Harvey Eppolito
ISBN: 978-1-60741-596-1

Chapter I

Food Safety of Products of Vegetable Origin

Adriano G. da Cruz[1], *Eduardo H. de M. Walter*[1], *Anderson de S. Sant'ana*[2,4], *Luz Maria Paucar-Menacho*[1,5], *Verônica O. Alvarenga*[4], *Jose A. F. Faria*[1] *and Maria Cristina Antun Maia*[3]

[1]Departament of Food Technology, State University of Campinas, Brazil
[2]Departament of Food and Experimental Nutrition, State University of São Paulo, Brazil
[3]Departament of Biochemical Engineering, Federal University of Rio de Janeiro, Brazil
[4] Department of Food Science, State University of Campinas, Brazil
[5]Department of Agroindustrial Engineering, National University of Santa, Perú

1. Introduction

Fruit and greens are traditional components of the Brazilian diet and their uneventful consumption has been stimulated in several countries, as the consumers perceive them as healthy, tasteful, convenient and fresh foods. They are vitamin sources, besides having compounds with antioxidant action, as lycopen, lutein and alpha-carotene that, at cellular level, hinder the accumulation of free radicals, minimizing the cancer occurrence (Fahrasmane et al., 2007). Williamson (1996) verified that an increase of consumption of leaf vegetables (cauliflower, broccoli) was related to a reduction of risk of developing cancer in the intestine and in the thyroid. Musgrove (2008) reports that the medium number of present portions of vegetables and fruit in England was 3.1 and an increase in the number of children ingesting five or more portions was observed (Musgrove, 2008). Another study performed in the United States reports that 55% of people believe that compounds naturally present in these foods may help to prevent diseases, being reported the consumers' preference for their ingestion (Childs and Poryzees, 1998). Consequently, the food industry, researches and consumers have been showing great interest in the antioxidant power of phlavonoids, anthocyanins and other present phytochemical compounds which can have protecting effect against cancer and cardiovascular diseases (Ness and Powles, 1997).

2. Food of Vegetal Origin as Vehicle of Food Poisoning

Virtually, any type of food is susceptible to become contaminated by pathogenic microorganisms, but this does not necessarily implicate occurrence of human diseases (Brackett, 1999). Some microorganisms can only cause diseases if ingested in high concentrations, as for instance, *C. perfringens*, or when they meet favorable conditions to develop and produce toxins, as *C. botulinum*, emetic *Bacillus cereus* or *Staphylococcus aureus*. However, in many cases the infective dose is relatively low. Consequently, the contamination of food and the survival of the pathogenic microorganism until the moment of consumption may implicate disease. In the transmission of viruses or parasites, for instance, it do not occurs the microbial development in foods (Harris et al., 2003). Besides that, it should be considered that, in most of the cases, the infective dose is dependent on the people's individual susceptibility (Institute of Food Technologists - IFT, 2000).

Despite several pathogenic microorganisms have been detected in a variety of fruit and greens, just some fresh products were involved in transmission of diseases. In the United States some large outbreaks associated with the consumption of melon, tomato, raspberry, lettuce, onion, alfalfa sprout and apple and orange juices happened (NACMCF, 1999). Between 1990 and 2003, foods of vegetal origin were responsible for 554 alimentary outbreaks, resulting in 28.315 cases, which correspond to 12% of the total of outbreaks and 20% of the registered cases. The most common item involved was salads containing several vegetables and alfalfa seeds, being registered prevalence of bacteria commonly found in food of animal origin, as *Salmonella* spp, *Campylobacter* spp and *E.coli* O157:H7 in 30% of the cases (Dewaal et al., 2006). Another survey between 1982 and 2002, with the exclusive objective of discriminating the sources of food poisoning outbreaks related to *E. coli* O157:H7 in the United States, identified that 21% of these were related to MPV, 74% occurring between the months of July to October and 34% being associated with lettuce (Rangel et al., 2005). Additionally, another survey done by the Centre for Disease Control – CDC identified 21 outbreaks (0.5%) cause by fruit juices between 1995 and 2005, which resulted in 1366 victims, 149 hospitalizations, 17 internments and one death. *Salmonella* was involved in 710 (52%) of the breaks and 95 (63%) of the internments. Apple juice was shown as vehicle of the outbreak in 10 (nearly 50%) of the total of outbreaks (Vojdani et al., 2008). Recently, fresh produce was pointed as the main food item associated with the occurrence of non-tpyphoidal Samonellosis cases in North Dakota, USA from 2000 to 2005, being responsible to 72.8% of the cases (Tumuhairwe et al., 2008).

Epidemiological studies evidence that the diseases transmitted by fruit and vegetables are transmitted by a variety of bacteria, viruses and parasites (NACMCF, 1999). Despite these organisms present a wide physiological variety, there is a common feature: their primary source is the enteric environment, in other words, they are found in intestinal tract and faecal material of human beings and animals. Exceptions include: *C. botulinum*, usually isolated from soil, aquatic environment and organic matter in decomposition; and *L. monocytogenes*, promptly isolated from human and animal faeces, as well as from agricultural and industrial environments (Harris et al., 2003).

In Brazil, there were no official estimates available about the prevalence or incidence of foodborne diseases associated with the consumption of fruit and vegetables. However, recent studies show an alarming situation: In São Paulo, Brazil, 61% of the samples of this vegetable analyzed registered populations of fecal coliforms above 10^2 CFU/g, whilst in Campinas, Brazil, this index only reached 3.2% of the total, with a mean population of 1.2 MPN/g, the positivity index oscillating according to the season of the year, being 62.5% in the summer and 12.5% in the winter (Porto and Elroa, 2001; Froder et al., 2007). In other research, Silva et al. (2007) evaluated the bacteriologic and parasitologic contamination in minimally processed, ready-to-eat vegetables available in supermarkets in the city of Porto Alegre. The mesophilic count ranged from $4.7x10^5$ to $1.6x10^8$ CFU/g ,while the psychrotrophic one ranged from $7.9x10^6$ to $2.7x10^8$ CFU/g. Total coliforms ranged from <3 to $\geq 2.4x10^4$ MPN/g and faecal coliforms from <3 to $1.1x10^4$ MPN/g. *Escherichia coli* was detected in eight samples. 15.3% of the samples presented oocysts of *Eimeria* spp; Dirt matter, such as insect body parts and young mites, was also found.

3. Sources of Contamination of Food of Plant Origin

The microbial contamination of vegetables is largely associated with surfaces of fruit and vegetables, as their internal layer is usually considered sterile. For this reason, leaf vegetables, which have larger superficial area, frequently have a higher degree of contamination (De Roever, 1998). There is a large probability for fruit and vegetables being contaminated by pathogenic microorganisms due to their exposure to a large variety of conditions which they are exposed during their growth, as reported by Table 1 (Madden, 1992). Usually, the earlier this happens in productive chain, it becomes more difficult the disinfection of the product, as there is a larger probability of the microorganism adhere to inaccessible places by the sanitizer, incorporated in bio films or internalized in the interior of the fruit or vegetable (Sapers,2001). The lack of a step of thermal death between the growth and the consumption also shows that pathogens introduced at any point of the processing line may be present when the product is consumed. For most of enteric pathogens the last sources are the animals and human beings' faeces. However, the specific way through which the product is contaminated are several, and include as much direct as indirect ways of transmission such animals, soil, water and human handling (De Roever, 1998).

Table 1. Sources of Microbial Contamination of Fruits and Vegetables

Irrigation water
Deficient cleaning and sanitization
Equipment
Inadequate use of manure
Wild animals
Washing water
Cross-contamination with processed product

Source: Madden, 1992

Actually, once the pathogen is introduced in product, there is no trustable and effective way of eliminating it and to face this situation the processors have to centralize efforts to (Fain, 1996):

(a) Keeping pathogens out of the processing plant, when they just buy them from suppliers who can supply safe products;
(b) Avoid contamination of the product through the uneventful set of cleaning and sanitization in all the processing plant, which will have its efficiency tested through random microbiological analysis of the environment;
(c) Reduce the microbial lead through washing with suitable concentrations of sanitizers;
(d) Reduce the growth of microorganisms through temperature and time control in order to avoid abuses of these parameters.

It is important to state that in processing plants of vegetal origin foods, the primary sources of contamination are the raw materials accepted and the contamination of the product along its productive process, which includes handlers, appliances/pieces of equipment and environment (Fain, 1996). The contamination of fresh fruit and greens is worrying, for, previously to their consumption, these products are not subjected to any kind of treatment, as boiling, which effectively destroys the vegetative cells of pathogenic microorganisms. This hazard can be enlarged in products minimally processed and in juices, whose processing typically involves human contact, water immersion and section (Brackett, 1999), while its distribution and commercialization require shelf life of several days (Nguyen-The Carlin, 1994). The prevention of fruit and greens contamination by physical, chemical and mainly biological hazards is a fundamental pre-requisite in safety warranty and quality of fresh products. However, even in the best conditions of production and processing, the contamination of fresh products is practically unavoidable (National Advisory Committee on Microbiological Criteria for Foods - NACMCF, 1999).

The contamination can increase during the processing or at domestic level, either by infected handlers, and either by the contact with water, work surfaces, packages or other contaminated environments. In the agricultural environment, the soil, water, animals and handlers are especially important in this contamination of fruit and vegetables (NACMCF, 1999). The fertilization of soil with manure or municipal bio solids (sewer) improperly steady is considered one of their main sources of contamination (International Fresh-Cut Produce Association, 1999). It has been a common practice in several countries, but it may have potential negative consequences for the product, as it may spread pathogens found in soil (Beuchatt, 2006).

The fecal contamination of soil may increase if there are no suitable sanitary installations in the vicinity of the production areas. There are several sources of water pollution, being the most common the direct ejectment of municipal bio solids in the watercourse and the lixiviation of the contaminated soil. The importance of the identification and control of potential sources of water contamination is enlarged, considering that the water used in agriculture is usually not treated. Besides the water quality, other factors as the kind of irrigation may influence the contamination of fruit and greens. The irrigation techniques which expose the plants to a direct contact with water, increase their probability of contamination (NACMCF, 1999). The wild or domestic animals and the plagues constitute another potential source of contamination of fruit and greens, either in agricultural environment, or either after the harvest. However, while the domestic animals can be avoided in production areas and handling of foods, the control of sylvan animals or plagues are limited (Harris et al., 2003).

The harvest is a critical step due to the potential of contamination through the contact of the hands with fruit and vegetables. The expansion of this contact varies according to the type of product and the technology applied in harvest and in some post-harvest operations. The good practices of personal hygiene are largely alleged and they should be associated with the rationalization of techniques of food handling, preventing the direct contact of the hands with fruit and greens (ICMSF, 1996). The gloves must be used in specific phases and by trained handlers. Other surfaces that which are used to manipulate fruit and vegetables at the moment of the harvest (equipment, appliances, and recipients) and in their transport should be projected and built in order to avoid depositions of filthiness and make easier their higienization.

The higienization of fruit and vegetables should be associated with the control of air contaminants, installations, equipment and appliances involved in this operation and in the subsequent phases of the processing. As the higienization typically do not remove or inactivate completely the pathogenic microorganisms present in raw material, the processing of a contaminated lot may result in contamination of the environment and of the processing surfaces (Vanetti, 2004). In this cycle of contaminations, the water, in liquid state or as ice, may be contaminated or be an important source of pathogenic microorganisms of fruit and vegetables. Water is largely used in the processing of most fruit and greens, and the contamination of these products can happen as much in rinse as in other operations, as refrigeration, transport, higienization or application of waxes and fungicides (IFT, 2000). Hence, the quality of raw material, fundamental condition for the safety of the final product, also involves prevention of several types of cross contamination.

The prevention and the control of the contamination of fruit and vegetables comes from the attempt of understanding the fundamental physical, chemical and environmental features of this ecosystem and allied to the effect of external interventions in the behaviour of the pathogenic microorganisms.

3.1 Physical Features

The vegetal epidermis is the primary barrier against microbial infections, insects and physical damages in fruit and greens. This structure is covered by hydrophobic multi layers which form the cuticle (1-15 μm of thickness) (Frank, 2001). The distribution of microorganisms in vegetal surface is related to the wetability of its surface. The difference of microbial adherence between the lettuce and the cabbage, for instance, it is partially attributed to differences in the power of retention of superficial water of these leaf vegetables or in the hydrophobicity of the layers of cuticle (Lund, 1992). The vegetal surface, in spite of being apparently flat, consists of an irregular structure. The microbial adherence and colonization are facilitated by pores (stomates and lenticels), irregularities (broken thricomas, cracks in cuticle) and superficial injuries (Frank, 2001). The adherence of microbial cells in vegetal surface and their localization in protecting structures can hamper their removal or increase their resistance to antimicrobial treatments (Burnett and Beuchatt, 2000). This situation may be worsen in products with large superficial area, as the vegetables (Lund, 1992).

The pathogenic microorganisms can survive in surfaces of fruit and greens, but their development is uncommon. This is partially attributed to the typical disability of pathogenic microorganisms in producing enzymes necessary to the degradation of the vegetal epidermis, which restrains the availability of nutrients and water (Harris et al., 2003). However, the development of the resident microbiota in vegetables may damage the integrity of the epidermis and change the pH of the media, increasing the probability of survival and development of pathogens. Wells e Butterfield (1997) detected *Salmonella* sp mainly in rotten products.

The possibility of survival and development of pathogenic microorganisms is considerably increased when the protecting barrier of the epidermis is disrupted. This disruption may occur in several ways: by incidental mechanical injuries; by animals; by microorganisms; and by intended sections, as in minimally processed fruit and vegetables. It exposes the internal vegetal tissues, transfers the microorganisms of the surface of the intact product for the internal tissues and releases the vegetal fluids from the injured cells (Harris et al., 2003).

3.2 Chemical Features

The surface of fruit and vegetables has a resident microbiota that normally subsists in enough amount of nutrient, including carbohydrates, proteins, mineral salts and humidity, arising from the vegetal exudation or from the environmental condensation. Several vegetables have their surface covered with tubular protuberances called thricomas. The thricoma glandules secrete chemical substances on the surface of vegetables which have antimicrobial activity and are repellent to insects. Other substances that come from the environmental pollution and from the agrochemical control may interfere on the resident microbiota and on the contaminant on the surface of vegetables (Spurr, 1994).

Some similar microorganisms are usually found in fruit and vegetables. However, the chemical composition of each kind of vegetable may be different from the contaminant and resident microbiota. In vegetables with pH close to neutral value, the bacteria are usually present in large abundance. Not so long ago, it was generally believed that fruit of high acidity and low pH presented a despicable risk. This consideration was based on the antagonist effect of acids and of pH over most of the bacteria. Despite these conditions prevent the development of many pathogenic microorganisms; the product may be contaminated with biological hazards in sufficient level to cause diseases. Some pathogenic microorganisms as *E. coli* (Goodson and Rowbury, 1989), *Listeria monocytogenes* (Kroll and Patchett, 1992) e *Salmonella* Typhimurium (Foster and Hall, 1991) may be adapted to conditions of acidity which would be normally lethal. Besides that, there are evidences that the development of pathogenic microorganisms in certain sublethal pH conditions may increase their virulence and initiate adaptive mutations which select strains more resistant to other stressing conditions (Archer, 1996).

3.2 Environmental Features

The environmental conditions in field are considered typically inhospitable for the survival and development of many microorganisms. This is partially attributed to the incidence of luminous radiation and to temperature and humidity fluctuations (Spurr, 1994). After the harvest, the behaviour of microorganisms, including the pathogenic ones basically depends on the temperature, humidity, atmosphere and intrinsic characteristics of the vegetable (Harris et al., 2003). The refrigeration is typically used to lag the breathing, the senescence, the darkening, the loss of humidity and the microbial development in fresh products (Seymour and Appleton, 2001). However, the microorganisms usually survive to low temperatures, and there are also those psychrotrophic ones which are able to develop under refrigeration, even at a slower speed than the one of room temperature. Some of these microorganisms are pathogenic, as strains of non-proteolytic *Clostridium botulinum*, *L. monocytogenes* and *Yersinia enterocolitica* (Parish et al., 2003). Another worrying microbial class in refrigerated products is the viruses. There are evidences that the enteric viruses are able to persist in different types of surfaces, poriferous or flat, for periods of more than 30 days, being observed more survival in the temperature of 4ºC than in 20ºC (Abad et al., 1994). A very common practice in laboratories that work with viruses is their preservation under frozen conditions (ICMSF, 1996). Despite that, the temperature control is critical for the safety of fresh products. The use of modified atmosphere packaging together with the refrigeration is still considered not technologically safe. As in refrigeration, this technique may favour the development of pathogenic microorganisms in detriment of the activity of other competitor microorganisms, in a way that the product does not present deterioration signs and be consumed (Harris et al., 2003). *Clostridium perfringens*, *C. botulinum* and *L. monocytogenes* are minimally affected by levels of CO_2 below 50%. High levels of O_2 (80-90%) stimulate the development of pathogenic microorganisms, as *E. coli* and *L. monocytogenes* (Amanatidou et al, 1999).

4. Hazards in Food of Plant Origin

4.1. Microbiological Hazards

Both fungi and bacteria grow well on the vegetables. However, bacteria typically grow faster than yeasts and molds in the neutral environmental of most vegetables. Hence, vegetables tend to select bacteria, which are then present in greater abundance.. Unlike vegetables, most fruits select for fungi. Fruits typically contain sufficient acidity to effectively restrict growth of many bacteria (ICMSF, 1996)

4.1.1 Bacteria

The pathogenic bacteria are particularly worrying in fruit and greens because they have the capacity of developing before the consumption of the fresh product (NACMCF, 1999), with the safe-conduct that in many cases it does not occur perceptible changes, even in relatively large populations. Yet the activity of a diversified microbiota may provide indication of temperature abuse and age of the product by means of deteriorations. Besides that, the pathogenic bacteria may be inhibited or even eliminated by the action of the competitor or antagonist microbiota, which is naturally found in fruit and greens (Schuenzel and Harrison, 2002). Consequently, specifications requiring a very low counting of bacteria may damage the safety of fresh products (Harris et al., 2003).

Additionally, for most bacterial species the question of the MID cannot be answered satisfactorily. Firstly, it must bem borne in mind that among consumers there are special risk groups, like small children, senior citizens, pregnant women and immunocompromised persons. Furthermore, there are various physiological factors that influence the MID, for example: the degree of stomach fluid acidity; the quantity of stomach contents; the intestinal flora; and last but not least, the immunological status of the person (Untermann, 1998).

However, high microbial load indicates unsuitable conditions of obtainment, processing or packaging of fruit and greens. Additionally, fruit and greens present propitious conditions for growth of pathogenic microorganisms with survival to lower values of pH. Penteado and Leitão (2004a, b) verified growth of *Salmonella Enteritidis* and *Listeria monocytogenes* in pulps of tropical fruit as melon, watermelon, papaya in several temperatures of storage, being observed that the low values of pH were not obstacles for the growth of pathogens and that the growth speed was proportional to the storage temperature used .Castillo et al.(2006) related the presence of *Salmonella* and *Shigella* sorovars in fresh squeezed orange juice sold in streets and small food service establishments. Both pathogens were found in oranges juices, fresh oranges and wiping cloth samples, besides high aerobic counts and >3.0 log UFC/mL *E.coli* counts. The total and fecal coliform groups and the detection of *E. coli* are commonly used for the evaluation of hygienic-sanitary quality of foods. However, the presence of coliform groups in fruit and greens is considered normal, once they make part of the natural microbiota of plants and cannot be associated with a fecal contamination. Hence, it is recommended the utilization of *E. coli*, the most valid indicator of fecal contamination (Kornack and Johson, 2001). But its presence, even in higher concentrations, does not necessarily mean that it has occurred fecal contamination. *E. coli* may develop in several ecological housings, including the processing environment, or becoming part of the resident microbiota of industry, especially when the higienization is unsuitable (Cox et al., 1988). Thus, one of the most important applications of the coliform groups and of the analyses of *E. coli* is in the evaluation of higienization programs of fruit and green, as well as of the hygienic conditions in the processing environments (Kornacki and Johson, 2001). Abadias et al.(2008) performed a survey of minimally processed fruits and vegetables and sprouts in some establishments in Lleida, Spain between 2005-2006 with the aim to check the microbial contamination. The highest mesophilic and psychotropic counts were observed in fresh-cut vegetables, while the lowest ones were observed in fruits; absence of pathogens were related at these samples. High incidence of *E.coli* (40%) was noted in sprouts.

4.1.2 Fungi

Fungi that are related to outbreaks are almost entirely, producers of mycotoxins. Thus, they should not be considered as threats to food security, but the products of their metabolism (Untermann, 1998). Particularly in the case of foods of plant origin, the fungi play key role in those ones which has low humidity and are kept stored for long periods, such as rice, wheat, flour and etc. .. In these products, they produce mycotoxins (toxic metabolites). Several mycotoxins are related to food of plant origin and in some cases, the plant and mycotoxin is very well established.. In case of minimally processed vegetables and fruits, the micoflora is dominated by *Cladosporium*, *Alternaria* and *Penicillium*, while *Geotrichium* is less common. Already Alternaria, Cladosporium, Penicillium and Phoma were the most common fungi isolated from sprouts (Tournas, 2005). Despite they are able to produce mycotoxines , there is a short time between processing and consumption (few days) and unfavourable conditions to fungal growth as low temperature and gas mixture in this packaging.

4.1.3. Viruses

The viruses do not develop in foods, for they need specific alive cells to replicate. However, there are evidences indicating that these microorganisms are resistant to a variety of adverse conditions, and they can remain in food for a period much superior to its shelf life and in enough quantity to cause disease. The presence of the enteric viruses in foods is attributed in large part to the human faecal contamination, once the human organism is their definite source of contamination (ICMSF, 1996). The viruses may be excreted in large quantity through the faeces (until 1011 particles of rotavirus per gram of faeces) of infected individuals for periods that may vary between several days and several weeks, depending on the virus and phase of infection (Koopmans and Duizer, 2004). An important source of these hazards is the infected people who present minimum or imperceptible clinical symptoms (asymptomatic hosts). It is known that the main excretion period of the A hepatitis virus is before the appearing of clinical symptoms (Koopmans and Duizer, 2004).

In a general way, viruses represent a potential hazard for foods of vegetal origin, which offer suitable conditions for their development. Croci et al. (2002) investigated the survival of hepatitis A virus in fresh-cuts. The highest quantity was detected for lettuce, being related a slight decrease after nine days, last day of the storage. Fennel presented similar behavior of the lettuce, although it showed a more expressive reduction while the carrot present one logarithm lower the quantities detected for the other vegetables. Leong et al. (2008) related the survival of SA11 rotavirus in fresh juices of ripe pineapples, papayas and honeydew melons.

4.1.4 Parasites

Parasites, among which *Entamoeba histolytic*a, the most known human parasite which can be transmitted by fruit and vegetables, are the responsible for amoebic dysentery or amebiasis. It has access to fruit and vegetables through human or animal contamination, use of polluted water and insects. As its cysts are promptly destroyed by chloration and seasoning, the best way to avoid it is keeping high sanitary standards (Willey, 1997). *Cyclospora* oocysts, pathogen emergent in the 1990' is an unicellular parasite that causes longstanding diarrhea. Its medium period of incubation is nearly a week and person to person contamination has not been reported. Monge and Chinchilla(1996) investigated the presence of Cryptosporidium spp. oocysts, fecal coliforms, and Escherichia coli at 640 samples from eight different vegetables used for raw consumption in Costa Rica. Cryptosporidium spp. oocysts were found in 5.0% (4 samples) of cilantro leaves, 8.7% (7 samples) of cilantro roots and 2.5% (2 samples) of lettuce samples. A 1.2% contamination rate was detected in samples of other vegetables (radish, tomato, cucumbers and carrot) and a positive linear correlation ($P < 0.05$) established between the presence of Cryptosporidium spp. oocysts and fecal coliforms and *E. coli.* In 1999, *Cyclospora* was involved in Canada, in Toronto in a dinner offered to 400 guests. 26% of the guests had positive results for the pathogen, and analysis showed that the strawberry ice-cream was the contamination vehicle (Sewell and Farber, 2001).

Giardia lambia is a flagellated protozoary which may also contaminate fruit and vegetables and may cause gastrointestinal complications, being similar to amebiasis either in symptoms, either in causes. It is estimated that 1,5 – 20% of Americans are hosts of this parasite, and the young people are the most susceptible ones. Raw fruit and vegetables, including lettuce and strawberries have been implicated in giardiasis outbreaks, and chlorinated water has not shown to be effective in the destruction of its eggs (Willey, 1997). Infections involving *G. lambia* may be acquired by person-to-person transmission or ingestion of water, ice or foods contaminated with faeces (Beuchatt, 1996*).*Although less common than other parasites *Ascaris lumbricoides* is also a potential problem in fruit and vegetables. The use of waters originated from excrements and organic fertilizers in the growth of minimally processed increases the risk of infections by this organism. Its eggs are very resistant to extreme conditions, including seasoning and chemical disinfectants and survive in storage for refrigeration temperatures for at least 20 years. Hence, techniques normally used in the minimum processing are improbable to destroy this microorganism (Willey, 1997).Between August 1999 and January 2001, samples of various fruits and vegetables obtained within Norway were analyzed for parasite detection. Neither *Cyclospora* oocysts nor Ascaris (or other helminth) eggs were detected on any of the samples examined for these parasites. However, of the 475 samples examined for Cryptosporidium oocysts and Giardia cysts, 29 (6%) were found to be positive. Of the 19 Cryptosporidium-positive samples, 5 (26%) were in lettuce, and 14 (74%) in mung bean sprouts. Of the 10 Giardia-positive samples, 2 (20%) were in dill, 2 (20%) in lettuce, 3 (30%) in mung bean sprouts, 1 (10%) in radish sprouts, and 2 (20%) in strawberries. Cryptosporidium oocysts and Giardia cysts were also detected in water samples concerned with field irrigation and production of bean sprouts (Robertson and Gjerde, 2001).

4.2 Chemical Hazards

The presence of residues of chemical substances – almost all of them pesticides – in food of plant origin destined to the human consumption constitute a large problem for public health in the present, as among the possible effects of these residues for the consumers there are problems of cancer, neurological, effects over the reproductive system and metabolism. This is result of the large variety of chemical molecules present in the structure of these compounds and their different forms of action, permeation and elimination, besides their different levels of noxiousness (Carinanos, 2005). Pasley and Skrzypczyk (2005), investigating the challenges involved in the consumption of fruit and greens among Canadian women, observed that although there were several benefits reported from the consumption of these foods, the interviewees were highly concerned with the presence of pesticides. Brewer and Rojas (2008) enumerating the American consumers' attitudes concerning to several topics of food safety, the presence of pesticides in foods was reason of concern of 50% of the interviewees.

The term 'pesticide' is used to describe any chemical agent that controls pests. The major classes of pesticides used in fruit and vegetable production are insecticides, herbicides and fungicides, although other types of pesticides such as moluscicides, bacteriocides, nematicides, acaricides, plant growth regulators and pheromones are also frequently used(Winter,2005). They are used at all stages of agriculture and food production beginning with pretreatment of fields (weed control) and housing (pest control), through crop (pest, weed and fungus control) and animal (pest control) treatments, to treatment of harvested food (pest and fungus control). In addition, pesticides used in crop production may contribute to subsequent animal exposure due to use of the crop as a feedstuff. Examples include organochlorine, organophosphorous and carbamate pesticides (O'Keeffe and Kennedy, 1998) Among the organic chemical hazards, pesticides are included in residuals chemical category: contaminants already present within or on a foodstuff resulting from previous exposure of ingredients or raw materials during food production, processing or packaging. (Ropkins and Beck, 2003).

The difficult in controlling the effects caused by the use of pesticides in foods is in the fact that this is an invisible contamination, and it is necessary an exposure time so that it is manifested through some visible symptom (ANVISA, 2006). Besides, their formulation has the presence of active ingredients or inert additives which provide nutrients for growth of bacteria. Guam et al. (2005) recovered Salmonella and *E.coli O157:H7* added to pesticide solution at 6 log UFC/mL from the leaves and fruit skin of sprayed tomato plants after a recommended day to harvest of one day.

A total of 722 million pounds lb (328 million kg) of pesticide active ingredients was estimated to be used in 2000, including 432 million lb (196 million kg) of herbicides and plant growth regulators, 90 million lb (41 million kg) of insecticides and miticides and 44 million lb (20 million kg) of fungicides. Estimated pesticide declined in 2001 to 675 million lb (306 million kg), including 433 million lb (197 million kg) of herbicides and plant growth regulators, 73 million lb (33 million kg) of insecticides and miticides and 42 million lb (19 million kg) of fungicides. Another major class of pesticides, nematicides and fumigants, accounted for an estimated 131 million lb (60 million kg) of active ingredient used in 2000 and 102 million lb (46 million kg) used in 2001(Winter,2005). Brazil was classified as the eighth country among the largest consumers of pesticides and the fourth largest market of pesticides of the world; in 2006 it represented the second largest pesticide consumer market in the world (Rodrigues, 2006). Through the Program of Residues Analysis in Foods (PRAF) elaborated by the Brazilian Sanitary Surveillance 6123 samples of fruit and vegetables were analyzed. It was observed that the largest problem is not at the levels that exceed the limit allowed by legislation which were found, but in the indiscriminate use of non authorized pesticides for the cultures. Strawberry (54.55%) and lettuce (46.46%) were the products with the largest indexes of non conformities, presenting residues above the minimum limits imposed by legislation (ANVISA, 2007).

It is important to understand that pesticide use does not necessarily imply pesticide residues. Many pesticides are applied prior to the planting and/or development of edible portions of the commodities while other pesticides may be sufficiently eliminated from a food crop prior to harvest (Winter, 2000).

The hazards to human healthy coming from the incorrect handling and longstanding exposure to pesticides make the concentration monitoring of these compounds an uneventful task of the health agencies in all over the world, independently of the degree of development of the country. In 1991, the USDA initiated its Pesticide Data Program (PDP) that collects, in cooperation with many state agencies, several thousand food samples that are analyzed for pesticide residues each year. In 1997, among fresh fruit and vegetables, samples of pears, potatoes, spinach, sweet potatoes, tomatoes, and winter squash were collected. Samples also were collected from six processed fruit and vegetable products: apple juice (ready-to-serve and concentrate), canned/frozen green beans, orange juice (ready-to-serve and concentrate), canned peaches, canned spinach, and frozen winter squash (Winter, 2000). At least one residue was detected in 70% of the fresh fruit and vegetable samples and in 45% of the processed fruit and vegetable samples. However, only four of the 6321 showed residues in excess of tolerance, although a total of 422 other presumptive violative residues were detected where tolerances for the detected pesticides were not established on these commodities (Winter, 2000). Saeed et al.(2001) investigated the presence of residues of chlorinated pesticides in Kuwait. Most of the fresh vegetables samples did not presented any pesticide residue, while 23.5% of fresh fruit ones contained detectable residues, being 13.6% positive for chlorinated pesticide residues. Poulsen and Andersen (2003) evaluated the exposure of the Danish populationto pesticides. Residues were found in 60% of the fruit samples but in only 18% of vegetables samples. Above the MRL were found 6% of all samples of fruits and 2% of vegetables samples, being registered a lower incidence at domestic products. Lesueur et al.(2007) investigated the residues of non polar and intermediate polarity pesticides in domestic and imported fruits and vegetables in Austria. 62% of the samples presentec detectable pesticide residues in 2004 and 54% in 2005, being 4% of the samples exceeded the MRL in 2004 and 7.7% in 2005.

The use of pesticides is an integrant part of contemporaneous agricultural practices, and it is related to search for lesser losses of agriculture products and the obtainment of larger production and consequently profit. However, important measures for minimizing the injures caused to health coming from its exposure pass mandatorily by the implementation of training programs concerning their use and handling in a safe way by the workmen, besides a constant inspection by the health agencies for the fulfilment of the present legislation, allied to periodic programs of monitoring to certify the quality of the products. In a HACCP system, due to the complexity and cost of the analysis, which are many times unavailable for most of the processors, a formal and written statement made by the producers certifying that only authorized pesticides for determined fruit or vegetable are used and are applied according to the determined instructions is used to accept the raw material of vegetal origin by the agro industrial plants.

4.3 Physical Hazards

The presence of physical hazards in fruits and vegetables, as any food, are related the foreign objects which can be introduced at many stages. Foreign objects may be defined as solid matter which is present in food, but which, whether of intrinsic or extrinsic origin, is undesirable. There are a number of major sources of foreign bodies in food that could be inadvertently present within raw materials, e.g., stones, woods or soil(Inteak,2004). According the FDA, a foreign object in food is categorized as a physical hazard is the following criteria are observed (a) there is clinical evidence of physical trauma or injury from its ingestion; b) the medical authorities recognize it as a potential ingestion hazard; (c) subsequent processing or intended use of the product does not eliminate or neutralize the product (Olsen and Zimmerman, 2003). The first condition is the most common physical hazard which is encountered in food products.

Physical hazards can be problematic to the agricultural production of food and may cause difficulties in the post-harvest activities of fruit and vegetable production. Consequently, they may be of concern to further processors and food manufacturers who use fruit and vegetables as raw materials, as well as ultimately to consumers(Early,2005). Soriano et al.(2005) studying the application of HACCP principles to salads served in university restaurant in Valencia, Spain related the existence of physical hazard at the raw vegetable receiving stage should be checked; they must be free of any foreign material. In this context, foreign body in fruits and vegetables can be safety issues and should be monitored inside a assurance quality system; typical injuries caused by them include choking, cuts and broken teeth: in extreme cases this may result in hospital treatment.

5. Prevention of Contamination in Fruit and Vegetables

A fundamental approach when elaborating a strategy to guarantee the safety of fruit and greens is the investigation of the nature of contaminants in productive chain. This phase must priorizated in detriment of analysis of the food, considering that the distribution of pathogenic microorganisms in foods is typically not uniform; their detection is infrequent and, when present, is usually in low concentrations (Brackett, 1999). Consequently, the studies of incidence are expensive and longstanding, being the generated information limited to a product of certain region and for a determined period of the year (Harris et al., 2003). Besides that, the determination of the pathogenic microorganism of largest significance or hazard index in food is presented as a high complexity task. Two additional questions arise: (I) the minimum dose of the microorganism able to cause the disease. Among the consumers, there are risk groups as children, pregnant, elder and imunocompromised hosts who present different physiological state which may influence the minimum quantity of viable cells that can cause the infection and (II) the dynamic of the microbial growth which is a dynamic phenomenon, subjected to different changes, being determined by several intrinsic and extrinsic factors and also food processing factors (Untermann, 1997). The understanding about the pathogenic microorganisms and their environmental purposes is limited, as it occurs a microbial evolution that is natural, and sometimes, catalyzed by human action.

6. Internalization of Pathogens in Foods of Vegetal Origin

The surface of fruit and vegetables grown in country and in orchards is natural habitat for microorganisms, bacteria, strains and fungi (Mendonca, 2005). The bacteria may intertwine in the vegetal tissues, being defined as internalized, which means allocated under the surface of the plant. These microorganisms cannot be removed with the washing of vegetables, and they are even protected against environmental stresses and cannot be inactivated by biocides and other superficial disinfectants (Bartz, 2006).

The internalization may occur via damaged tissues in surface of vegetables, by water contaminated in fields or in the post-harvest process of vegetables in washing phase. The internalization of bacteria causes losses in the post-harvest process and damages the microbiological safety of fruit and vegetables (Mendonca, 2005). This becomes a concern with the minimum processed vegetables, and fruit and fresh vegetables, because for the sanitization of these products techniques and products for surface sanitization are used, and these decontamination methods of surface are not effective to eliminate the pathogenic bacteria infiltrated in the vegetal tissues. Thus, the prevention of infiltration in fresh products is crucial to control the internalization of pathogens and to improve the microbiological safety and the shelf-life of fruit and vegetables (Mendonca, 2005).

Buchanan et al. (1999) studied the susceptibility of apples to contamination by immersion water. When the warm apples were submerged in colder water contaminated by *E. coli* O157:H7, in the same way that happen in the processing operations, where immersion tanks are not kept in a hygienic way, the pathogenic occasionally internalized. These results confirmed that 6% of the warm apples are submerged in water colder than the fruit; this temperature gradient opens grooves that make easier the internalization of pathogens into the interior of the fruit.

The infiltration of bacteria in warm fruit immerged in cold water can be explained by the gas law; as the temperature of fruit and vegetables is lesser, the gases contract the tissues, reducing the internal pressure. The reduction of pressure together with the atmospheric pressure produce an internal balance and this allows the water infiltration (Bartz, 2005).

The survival and growth of bacteria internalized in fruit and vegetables are influenced by several factors, including the type of bacterium, physiochemical characteristics of fruit and vegetables, and also of the post-harvest process and the storage conditions (Mendonca, 2005).

The internalization of bacteria of fruit and vegetables damage the shelf life and the microbiological safety of these products. The adherence of bacteria in fruit and vegetables may cause their infiltration by washing water or even by open ducts naturally through injuries on the vegetal surfaces. The bacterial infiltration is affected by temperature of the washing water, by hydrostatic pressure, by surfactants and the type of cooling system used in the post-harvest process. The infiltration of bacteria occurs mainly when the warm fruit is immerged in water. This negative differential of temperature makes possible the contraction of the vegetal tissues, permeabilizating where water penetrates the tissues. For the prevention of the internalization of bacteria techniques of the good agricultural practices are applied together with the temperature control and hydrostatic pressure during the post-harvest process.

7. Food Safety

Worldwide dictionaries distinguish between safety and security. Some interpret safety as an active form of safety and security is the passive form to assure safety. Connected to agricultural products, these two concepts have even more notation. Food security is regularly used in humanitarian actions, where we help the underdeveloped and those who need help. This means that supplies will contain quality foodstuffs that are nutritious, safe and acceptable culturally and ethnically. Food safety is defined as an assurance that food will not cause harm to the consumer when it is prepared and/or eaten according to its intended use (Raspor and Jevsnik, 2008).

Food safety is a result of several factors: legislation should lay down minimum hygiene requirements; official controls should be in place to check food business operators′ compliance, and food business operators should establish and operate food safety programs and procedures based on the HACCP principles (Raspor and Jevsnik, 2008).

8. Food Safety for Food of Plant Origin

In products of vegetal origin, food safety is only meaningful if considered in a wide aspect of all productive chain, from field to table. In this context, the rural producer has to be based on good agricultural practices (GAP), the industry has to based on good manufacturing practices (GMP) and the sectors of transport and distribution have to control the critical points and the consumer has to prepare the food in a hygienic and responsible way, according to the instructions written on the label. Hence, it is considered an indispensable and mandatory practice for the adoption of the HACCP system in an effective way, the previous implementation of these two quality systems: Good Agricultural Practices (GAP), Good Manufacturing Practices (GMP), both allied to the Standing Operating Procedures (SOP), as shown in figure 1.

Topics covered by this assurance quality systems include microbiological hazards (*E. coli*, *Salmonella*, *Campylobacter*, *Listeria* etc.), nutritional hazards (fat consumption, obesity levels), environmental hazards (chemicals naturally occuring in foods (ingredients); and food composition hazards (Barendsz, 1998).

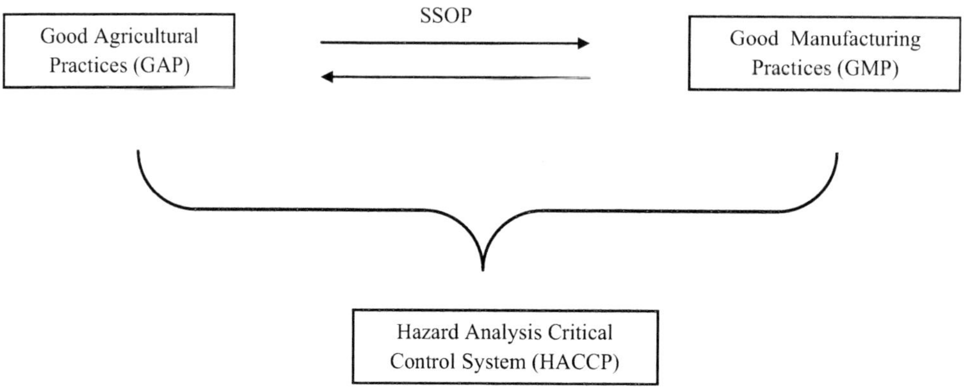

Figure 1. Food Safety Systems for Food of Plant Origin

9. Hazard Analysis and Critical Control Point (HACCP)

The hazard analysis critical control point (HACCP) system was originally developed for the US space programme as a means of making safe food for astronauts. It is now recommended as the best way to make safe food products, by the Codex Alimentarius Commission of the Food and Agriculture Organization (FAO) of the United Nations (UN) as well as the governments of many nations and food industry representative bodies (Early, 2005).

It involves the systematic assuring of all the phases involved in processing of foods, since table until the consumer, and their identification, which are critical concerning food safety and have shown to be extremely efficient in these purposes (Willock et al., *1994*): Aramouni et al. (1996) obtained meaningful reduction of mesophiles, psychrophiles, and total coliforms microorganisms in pieces of equipment and meaty products; Almeida et al. (1999) obtained reduction of 4,0, 3,0 and 4,0 log cycles in counting of mesophiles in infantile formulas, appliances and handlers respectively, besides the total elimination of *Salmonella* in fresh tomatoes after the adoption of the HACCP. It is demanded as mandatory part of the new measures destined to increase the safety of juices, due to food outbreaks transmitted by juices having as etiologic agent *E. coli* O157:H7; the process is used in industrial plant and has to avoid biological contamination and result, mandatorily, in a reduction of 5 log cycles in the population of the target pathogen, which is usually *E. coli* O157:H7 or *Salmonella* (Al-Taher and Knutson, 2004; Vojdani et al., 2008). It identifies the potential avenues of contamination; establishes control measures to eliminate or minimize these hazards; monitors and documents the effectiveness of the program. This system provides a more specific and critical approach to the control of the hazards than achievable by traditional inspection and quality control procedures (International Fresh-Cut Produce Association, 1999).

The HACCP program developed must be appropriate for each processing facility and for each product made at that facility. Instead of relying on finished product testing, regulatory inspectors or consumer complaints, the processors will have their own continuous problem-solving system (Al-Taher and Knutson, 2004).

Although the concept of HACCP can be translated for the management of quality factors not associated with food safety, HACCP itself should be used only for food safety management. HACCP systems should not be corrupted for the management of both food safety and non-food safety aspects of quality (Early, 2005). The HACCP plans for food of plant origin are well established and have been used successfully by processors for years, being based on the same seven principles and risk categories common in the control of meat, poultry and fish (Cruz, Cenci e Maia,2006a). These principles are conducted in the following order:

- Principle 1: Conduct a hazard analysis.
- Principle 2: Determine the critical control points (CCPs).
- Principle 3: Establish critical limit(s).
- Principle 4: Establish a system to monitor control of the CCP(s).
- Principle 5: Establish the corrective action to be taken when monitoring
- indicates that a particular CCP is not under control.
- Principle 6: Establish procedures for verification to confirm the HACCP system is working effectively.
- Principle 7: Establish documentation concerning all procedures and records appropriate to these principles and their application.

A critical control point (CCP) is a point, procedure, in a food processor which a control measure can be applied and at which control is essential to reduce an identified food hazard to an acceptable level(Al-Taher and Knutson, 2004). In fruit and vegetable production CCPs are likely to concern, for example, activities involving checking the concentration and application rates of pesticides or removing physical contaminants from produce. When applying hazard control measures at CCPs it is important not to incorporate into the HACCP plan activities that should be dealt with by GAP. For instance, it may be thought that the activity of calibrating sprayers constitutes a CCP (Early, 2005).

The HACCP system centres its attention on critical operations in which control is essential, differing from the traditional inspection control, directed mostly at factors of an aesthetic nature or attending norms that frequently have no significance with respect to public health. In this way, one avoids the false sensation of safety frequently associated with inspections, in which dangerous practices are frequently not detected during the brief infrequent visits(Cruz, Cenci and Maia, 2006a). Once developed, the HACCP procedure should be implemented quickly and with minimum disruption to relevant activities. Under normal conditions, reviews of production practices and associated documents acts as an assurance that it has been correctly adhered to (Ropkins and Beck, 2004).

The growers of fruit and vegetables may independently recognise the benefits to be gained from the implementation of HACCP within their businesses, but such a requirement may inevitably be processors with whom they and the supermarkets do business (Early, 2005).

10. Prerequisite Programs

The HACCP system has been indicated as one of the most effective ways to guarantee high quality and safe food, from a human health point of view. However, its success and effectiveness in preventing foodborne diseases and risks to consumer health depend on the correct application of prerequisite programs, which include safety infrastructure: the ''Good manufacturing practice'' and ''Sanitation standard operational procedures'' (GMP/SSOP) (Roberto et al., 2005)

Prerequisite programs include elements previously, described as good manufacturing practices (GMP), for e.g., cleaning, operator and environmental hygiene, plant and building design and preventive manutence. What is new to many companies is the concept of formalizing pre-requisite programs alongside HACCP to control general hygiene and quality issues, allowing the HACCP plan to concentrate on controlling significant hazards (Wallace and Williams, 2001).

They are not part of the formal HACCP system. They frequently function across product lines and are often managed as facility-wide or company-wide programs rather than being product or process specific, as is the case with HACCP systems. Prerequisite programs can include objectives other than food safety, and it may not be easy to associate performance of a prerequisite program element, e.g., pest control or chemical storage programs, with specific production lost or batches (Sperber et al., 2001).

Deviations from compliance with a prerequisite program usually do not result in action against the product, while in the HACCP sytem it is possible what is a key consideration that distinguishes control points at the former and critical control points in at the latter. If a prerequisite program is not conducted adequately, then the hazard analysis may be in error and the HACCP plan may be inadequate. If the HACCP team cannot depend on consistent control of the prerequisite program, then additional critical control points(CCPs) may be need to be added to the HACCP plan, increasing its complexity; in short, reliance on well developed and consistently performed prerequisite programs can simplify the HACCP plan(Sperber et al., 1996). Wallace and Williams (2001) related a dry good mixing operator with 600 CCPs. The inclusions of critical control points in HACCP which are not true CCPs can cause problems in practice.

The HACCP system only hás CCPs. Using Other terms as critical points, critical controls, quality control points within the HACCP plan simply serve to confuse and to control food safety (Wallace and Williams, 2001). Mortimore (2000) proposes a scheme

(Figure 2) to demonstrate both (prerquesite programs and HACCP system) may be managed in a quality system.

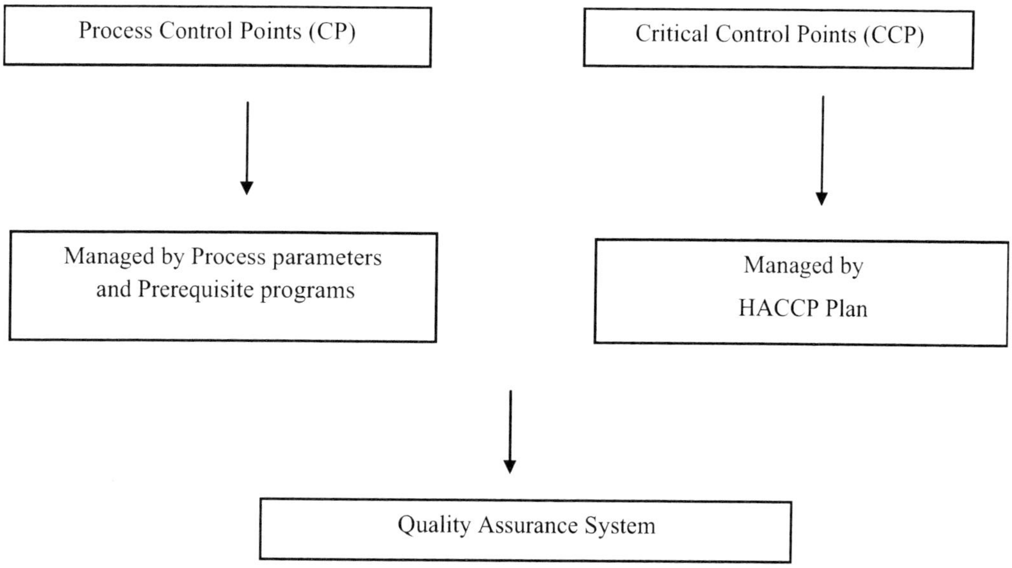

Source : Motirmore, 2000
Figure 2. Differentiation between Process Control Point (CP) and Critical Control Point (CCP)

By giving good control of basic principles of food handling, prerequisite programes can support HACCP effectively and the resulting streamlined HACCP plans can be easier to manage. In addition, the prerequisite programmes maybe a useful starting point with companies who have a longer way to achieve HACCP (Wallace and Williams, 2001). In fact, an effective result may be achieved if the prerequisite programs and HACCP work simultaneously: the hazards being managed by the latter and the topics related to hygiene/GMP managed by the former. That way, there will be small probability of shifting the focus HACCP system from its main purpose, the CCPs (Wallace and Wiliams, 2001). Food processors who adopted the PRPs before the HACCP system showed a significant improvement in sanitary-hygienic quality and, consequently, an increase in the level of safety at their lines, evidenced by the elimination of pathogens and the reduction of total microbial load (Tomé et al., 2000; Soriano et al., 2002).

11. Good Agricultural Practices (GAP)

Good agricultural practices are 'general procedures to reduce hazards related to product safety at field level during the operations that precede their processing, such as growth, development, harvest and storage, have to be established having as basis the risks associated with fruit and vegetables and the data available in literature (De Roever, 1998). As the Good

Manufacturing Practices (*Good Manufacturing, GMP)* the BPAs are considered a prerequisite program for implementation of a HACCP plan at field level.

In fact, the importance of a suitable level of safety in obtainment of raw material of vegetal origin expressed by the implementation of a quality warranty system as the GAPs, minimizes the chances of there being a processed product that may be a risk for the consumer's health. Kokkinakis et al. (2007) investigated the microbiological quality of tomatoes and pepper produced under AGRO 1 and 2-2, a GAP program implemented in greenhouses at Ierapetra, Crete, Greece: absence of *Listeria monocytogenes* and low counts of *Escherichia coli* was observed. Any change in the microbial quality of vegetables produced did not change significantly between the steps of growing and harvest, indicating stable hygiene. The spoilage bacteria *E. coli* and *S. faecalis* were not found in all 18 water samples.

Several researches have been conducting to identify the level of knowledge and adoption of GAPs from the farm processors.Wright et al(2000) related implications toward production of apple cider due to Viginia producers′ food safety practices. It was noted presence of animals in adjacents field in 54% of the farms beind still related the use of damaged fruit for production of cider for 37.5% of the producers. 37% use sanitizer after the washing of the fruits and the pasteurization step is just performed by 22% of the producers. However, although 2% include microbiological test at the finished cider and include expiration date on processed product label, the adoption of HACCP is considered by 67% of them.

Two interesting surveys towards GAPs adoption were conducted in New England, USA. Firstly, Cohen et al (2005) investigated the grower practices of fresh fruit and vegetables. It was observed use of non-composted manure by 22%, being one third of them store it for less than six months before applying it; 97% are able to prevent livestock and poultry from fields and 90% wash the harvest and sotrage containers " sometimes. The authors also related records of pesticides in 78% of the growers, besides records on packing or processing dates, field of origin and worker training by 25-35%. The daily cleaning of packaging equipment and checking the temperature refrigeration was related by 79% and 85%, respectively. However, just 14% used sanizer in the wash water. Overall, good performance towards GAPs adoption was observed. The second survey was performed by Pivarnik et al(2006). They evaluated of level of knowledge towards GAPs of home gardeners in New England:topics associated with safety of the produce, its association with pathogenic bacteria, use of manure and compost , water safety and washing presented low scores at the survey. Additionally, more than 50% of the questions were either answered incorrectly or without indication that the respondent did not know the answer. Jackson et al. (2007) performed a written survey on GAPs at growers and packers in some states of the USA. The adoption of this it affect positively the existence of toilete facilits in the field " most of the time" or " always" by the growers beside provision of adequate facility proper hand washing for workers in the field. Another valuable finding is the positive influence of GAP under provision of hygiene-specific worker training and the receiving of educational materials. Age and years farm of respondent and size of the farm did not affect GAPs awareness.

In the only research performed in South America, Cruz et al(2006c) evaluated the adoption of GAPs in a produce plan in São Paulo, Brazil. Some of critical points detected at the inspection were: absence analyses of the irrigation water and soil for the identification of heavy metals and pesticide residues, use of water without sanitizers to wash the harvest and storage equipments Besides, no formal procedure specifying norms of hygiene for the workers to follow when handling the produce were found and inexistence of previous training about food microbiology. Total traceability of the process was also observed. In a overall way, low scores in all blocks of the GAP checklist was related.

Izumi et al. (2008) identified on-farm sources of microbial contamination of persimmon fruit in Japan during its growing and harvesting. Samples of agricultural water, pesticide solution,soil and weeds besides several utensilis were collected. High levels of bacteria and fungi were found in soil or weeds. Microbial load of pesticide solution and agricultural water were very similar, and the predominan fungi isolated in the fruit were molds. No patoghen was detected. Weeds, plastic harvest baskets and cointainers appeared to be potential sources of fruit contamination at harvest stage, as the same bacteria were detected in the fruit and enviromental sample.

The principal objective of GAP is the management of agricultural resources to fulfill the human needs of agriculture while, at the same time, (1) protecting the environment and preventing pollution, (2) maintaining and enhancing the quality of the soil such that food production remains sustainable, (3) maximizing the welfare of animals in food production systems, (4) maintaining and enhancing the amenity value of the land and landscape, and (5) promoting conditions that restore and enhance biodiversity (Early, 2005).

Topics related to BPAs include the antecipation of sources and places in which the product may be contaminated, avoiding or minimizing the existent risks; existance of documented procedures in every phase to assure the product safety, and in many cases it is only necessary to meet the present legislation, as the building of hygienic-sanitary installations for the workmen, the use of organic fertilizaers which were sujected to composting for reduction of microbial load (Pabrua, 1999). De Roever (1998) reinforces this idea when he states the establishment of documented protocols related to irrigation water, use of fertilizers, hygien, appliances, people and transport.

One of the largest concerns in the concerns in safety of the product of vegetal origin consists in the quality of the irrigation water, being common the conclusion that it has many times high level of enteric bacteria and viruses. Evidence that contaminated irrigation water may be a source of foodborne pathogens on fruit and vegetables can be found in epidemiological investigations of food poisoning outbreaks (Steele and Odumeru, 2004).

Protozoas can also contaminate the product, being this level of contamination related to the form of irrigation and the type of product; the largest level is related with leaf vegetables that have superficial areas and structural characteristics that make easier the microbial adherence. (De Roever, 1998). Abdul–Rauof et al. (1993) found the presence of *Escherichia coli O157:H7* in chopped lettuce, associating as cause of its presence the possible contamination of the growth water. Techniques of irrigation that subject the plant to a direct contact with contaminated irrigation water (irrigation through spray) increase the risk of contamination of the product in detriment with the irrigation through depth. Solomon et al (2002) studied the transmission of *E. coli 0157:H7* in lettuce subjected (64 in total) to irrigation through spray (32) and through surface (32), obtaining a larger survival of the pathogen in the first case, with 29 positive cases (91%, survival for a period of 20 subsequent days to the treatment) in detriment to the second one where 6 positive results were registered (19%). Treatment with 200 ppm of chlorine for 1 minute did not eliminate the pathogen. Pabrua (1996) reinforces this idea when he emphasises the large quantity of applications that water has in operations at field level: washing and cooling of the product, application of pesticides, irrigation, among others and thus, it is rather important the monitoring of its quality through periodic microbiological analysis and the total knowledge about the source of water to be used in several operations. Another potential source of pathogenic bacteria in agricultural environment that may reach the water used in the process is the presence of domestic or wild animals, as reports of *Salmonella* sp have been isolated of intestinal features of most animals of hot and cold blood (De Roever, 1998).

Recente study relates that a hydroponic tomato farm which operated under GPAs, it was for two eventual natural events: a water runoff and presence of wid animais inside it. It was registered presence of *E.coli* and *Salmonella* in tomatoes, water puddles feces of local wild and farm animals. Same sorotype of the later were isolated from tomatoes, opossums and mice, suggesting the importance of these animals as vehicle of pathogens (Orozco et al., 2008).

Guidelines governing the microbial quality of irrigation water vary considerably between countries and between groundwater, surface water and human wastewater sources of water; however is commun to stipulate counts of total coliforms, fecal coliforms, *E. coli*, fecal streptococci and nematode eggs as the microbial indicators most commonly used by water quality guidelines to dictate irrigation water quality. They are among the strictest, reflecting the high numbers of human pathogens present intreated wastewater. Differences among them reflect widespread uncertainty the actual risk of disease transmission from pathogens in irrigation water and economic restrictions on avaiable water quality; alhotugh high quality is always desirable, in some countries the economic costs associated with his treating is prohibitive (Steele and Odumeru, 2004).

Equally critical in BPAs are the existence of suitable sanitary installations for the field workers. It is indispensable the existence of clean and private installations higienically built and easily accessed by people who deal with the product, as well as clear instructions for its use and periodic training programs in suitable language to assure the maximum efficiency of the operation (Pabrua,1996). The handlers as potencial source of transference of pathogens in minimum processed vegetables, mainly if they have poor higienic-sanitary practices; the training programs are highlighted as the main challenges found by processors due to their cultural educational differences (Hurst,1995). As animals, the handlers who have poor hygienic-sanitary practices may be hosts for enteric pathogens and they represent a contamination source of the product as they handle it (De Roever,1998).

The use of unsuitable fertilizing practices also have to be taken into consideration according to *International Fresh-Cut Produce Association* (1999) and composting practices have to be extremely monitored so that the elimination of pathogens has been reached. Beuchat (1996) reported that the survival of *E. coli O157:H7* using bovine faeces as vehicle in lettuce under temperature of 4°C was of until 15 days, even with the initial load of 1 to 10 CFU/g.

Although it was observed the existence of the composting process, with specific place and far from plantations, the monitoring of this practice is crucial for the safety of the process. Droffner and Briton (1995) report the survival of *Salmonella* and *E. coli* for the minimum of 59 days in composted fertilizer kept at 60°C. The potential reduction of contamination of minimum processed vegetables implicates in adopting rigid methods of composting and storage periods of 60 days in summer and 90 days in winter before the application in the field (Howard and Gonzalez, 2001).

Equally important is the correct handling of pesticides to be used in contact with the product; just pesticides registered and authorized by official agencies have to be used, otherwise they can be a sorce of contamination of the product. The efficiency of this operation is reached when the establishment of clear instructions of handling, training of people who are going to have contact with the substances and registers of application, besides the existence of a responsible qualified technician to follow all the process (International Fresh-Cut Produce Association, 1999).

Although HACCP is not an integral part of GAP, it operates in conjunction with GAP and in the case of agricultural enterprises, GAP provides the foundation for HACCP. The value of GAP to HACCP is found significantly in the way it ensures that critical and prerequisite requirements are established such that HACCP systems can then be implemented and operated effectively and, importantly, without complication and unnecessary costs (Early, 2005).

12. Good Manufacturing Practices (GMP)

GMP covers key areas in the food processing environment (Inteak, 2004):

- Premises: site location, design and maintence; equipment construction, design and maintence, including control of services and calibration; cleaning schedules for the site, plant and equipment.
- Personnel: control of staff, visitors and contractors; protective clothing rules; jewellery policy and training procedures.
- Product: approved supplier scheme; raw material specifications including packaging; finished product specifications; storage and delivery of raw materials finished products; traceability system and product recall procedure.

Figure 3 shows elements normally covered by a GMP program. Success in the implantation of GMP depends on managerial support, specialization and motivation of the personnel, provision of resources and divulgation of the programme. Industries that have adopted the GMP programme have obtained the following results, amongst others (Cruz, Cenci and Maia, 2006a):

- Better quality, safer products, decrease in incidence of consumer complaints;
- Better, more agreeable, cleaner and safer working environment ;
- Greater employee motivation and productivity and improved psychological conditions.

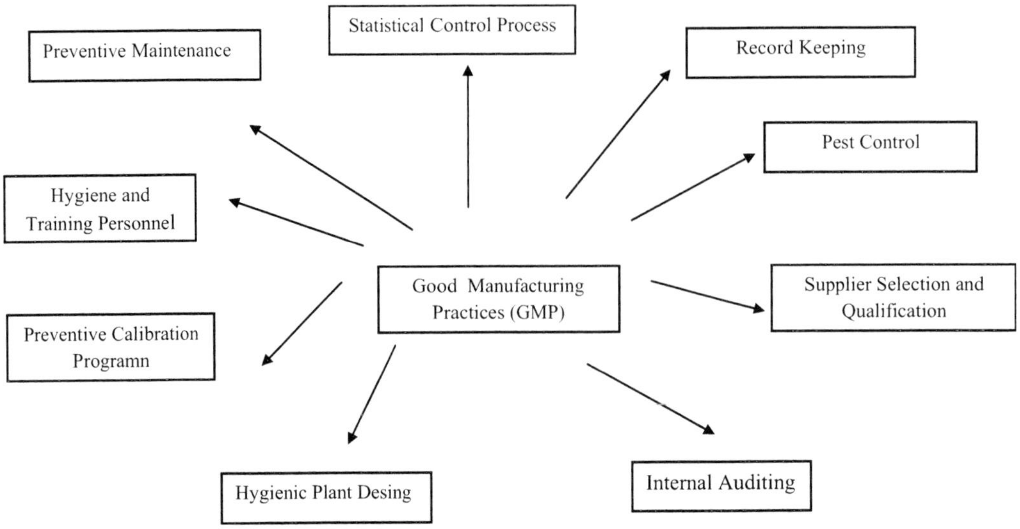

Figure 3. Elements of a GMP Program

The adoption of GMP in a production unit of food of plant origin, including fresh-cut products, follows the norms traditionally used in other food industries, although specificities related to the process according to the type of product being produced should be respected. In general terms the following steps are fundamental in a good manufacturing practices implementation programme for products of this type: control of the operations as expressed by the temperatures of the processing plant; control of the water using in product washing and sanitization; contact time and concentration of the sanitizer used in the process; sanitation programme for the cutting utensils used; personal hygiene of the handlers and of the air in the processing line; raw material inspection, which frequently requires the existence of a metal detector; prevention of cross contamination; control of final product storage temperature; pest control and instrument calibration programme. It is important to emphasize that it must be developed according to the reality of the processing unit and that special attention should be paid to the washing-sanitization binomial and the quality of the water used (Cruz, Cenci and Maia, 2006b).

Cruz, Cenci and Maia (2006b) evaluated a Brazilian produce line was evaluated according to prerequisite programs compliance. Several failures were detected in the GMP auditing and presence of pathogens and microbial groups were related - range from <3 to>16 MNP/100 mL and 7-2400 MPN/cm^2 for total and fecal coliform at the water processing and equipments/utensils, respectively). *S. aureus* was not detected on the handlers, while *E. coli* was present on them and absent at the water processing.

13. Sanitation Standard Operation Procedure (SSOP)

One of the prerequisites of HACCP is the development of SSOPs to address nom-specific food safety issues (Ropkins and Beck, 2003). Like GMP, sanitation standard operating procedures (SSOP) are also included in the pre-requisite programs category. They play complete description of the specific and common activities required to maintain the utensils free of pathogenic microorganisms and with the deteriorative flora minimized, consequently avoiding contamination of the food when in contact with these utensils and installations. Contamination occurs when biological, chemical or physical agents present in the processing environment are incorporated into the food during handling (Setiabuhdi et al., 1998).

The SSOP is the complete description of specific necessary activities to keep the installations and appliances free from pathogenic microorganisms and with the deteriorating microbiota minimized, which consequently prevents the contamination of food when in contact with these appliances and installations. The contamination occurs when biological, chemical or physical agents present in the processing environment are incorporated to the foods during their handling (Setiabuhdi et al., *1*998).

SSOP is a plan projected to prevent direct and indirect contamination of food products. It should include (Giese, 1991).

- A description of all the operational procedures for sanitization administered by the establishment:
- The specification and frequency of the procedures.
- Identification of the individual(s) responsible for the implementation and monitoring of the SSOP
- The signature and date of the individual with authority and implementation when adopted or modified.

As a general rule, they should not be included in the company HACCP plan, since the former control food safety risks associated with the plant environment (for example, installation maintenance and employee hygiene), whereas HACCP is effectively applied to the risks related to the step by step characteristics of product processing. The following central directives of SSOPs have been raised, considering the potential sources of contamination (Figueredo, 1999):

- Cross contamination of raw to cooked products, for example by surface contact with contaminated foods.
- Contact of product with non-potable water (e.g., condensation on exposed products) or other insalubrious substances.
- Contact with non-food substances (e.g. pesticides)
- Contact with substances transported by air.
- Handler diseases or inadequate hygiene.

- Foreign bodies in the food.
- Pests.

SSOPs are fundamental to quality assurance in food of plant origin processors, since they create registers of the fundamental activities in the control of the innocuousness of the process, guaranteeing success in the standardization of the activities and providing conditions for traceability if some abnormality occurs. They should thus be implemented together with the GMP programme. However, as with all quality assurance programmes, it is important to mention that a technician should manage their implementation with knowledge in food science and microbiology (Cruz, Cenci and Maia, 2006b). They should be performed using a simple and understanding language, through previous training with the employers.

References

Aamanatidou, A.; Smid, E. J. and Gorris, L. G. M. (1999). Effect of elevated oxygen and carbon dioxide on the surface growth of vegetable-associated micro-organisms. *Journal of Applied Microbiology*, 86, 429-38.

Abad, F. X.; Pinto, R. M. and Bosch, A. (1994). Survival of enteric viruses on environmental fomites. *Applied and Environmental Microbiology*, 60, 3704-3710.

Abadias, M.; Usall, J.; Anguera, M.; Solsona, C. and Vinas, I. (2008). Microbial quality of fresh, minimally processed fruit and vegetables and sprouts from retail establishments. *International Journal of Food Mi*crobiology, 123, 121-129.

Abdul-Rauof, U.M.; Beuchat, L.; and Ammar, M.S.(1993). Survival and growth of *Escherichia coli* O:157:H7 on salad vegetables. *Applied Environmental Microbiology*, 59, 1999 –2006.

Agência Nacional de Vigilância Sanitária.(2006). Pesticides residues in food. *Revista de Saúde Pública*, 40, 361-363.

Agência Nacional de Vigilância Sanitária.(2007). Programa de Análise de Resíduos de Agrotóxicos em alimentos (PARA). Available in: htpp//: www.anvisa.gov.br

Almeida, R.C.C.; Matos,C.O. and Almeida, P.F. (1999). Implementation of a HACCP system for on-site preparation of infant formula. *Food Control,* 10,191-187.

Al-Taher, F; Knutson, K.(2004). Overview of the FDA Juice HACCP Rule. *Food Protection Trends*, 24, 222-238.

Aramouni, F. M.; Boyle, E. A. E. and Vogt, L.R. (1996). Introduction to the Hazard Analysis Critical Control Point (HACCP) Concept in a Small Meat- Processing Plant. *Dairy , Food and Environmental Sanitation*, 16, 431-439.

Archer, D. L. (1996). Preservation microbiology and safety: evidence that stress enhances virulence and triggers adaptive mutations. *Trends in Food Science and Technology*, 7, 91-95.

Bai, L.; Yang, Y.; Zhao, S. and Gong, S. (2007). Implementation of HACCP system in China: a survey of food enterprises envolved. *Food Control*, 18, 1108-1112.

Barandsz, A.W. (1998). Food safety and total quality management. *Food Control*, 9, 163-170.

Bartz, J. A. (2006). Internalization and Infiltration. In: Microbiology of Fruits and Vegetables. Taylor and Francis, 2006. Chapter 3, 75-94.

Beuchat, L.R. (1996). Pathogenic microorganisms associated with fresh produce *Journal of Food Protection*, 59, 204-216

Beuchat, L.R. (2006). Vectors and conditions for preharvest contamination of fruits and vegetables with pathogens capable of causing enteric diseases. *British Food Journal*, 108, 38-53.

Brackett, R. E. (1999). Incidence, contributing factors, and control of bacterial pathogens in produce. *Postharvest Biology and Technology*, 15, 305- 311.

Brewer, M.S and Rojas, M. (2008). Consumer attitudes toward issues in food safety. *Journal of Food Safety*, 28, 1-22.

Buchanann, R.L.; Edelson, S.G.; Miller, R.L. and Sapers, G.M. (1999). Contamination of intact Apples after immersion in an Aqueous Environment Containing *Escherichia coli* O157:H7. *Journal of Food Protection*, 62, 444-450.

Burnett, S. L. and Beuchat, L. R.(2000). Human pathogens associated with raw produce and unpasteurized juices, and difficulties in decontamination. *Journal of Industrial Microbiology and Biotechnology*, 25, 281-287.

Castillo, A.; Villlaruel-Lopez, A.; Navarro-Hidalgo, V.; Martínez-Gonzalez, N.E.and Torres-Vitela, M.R. (2006). *Salmonella* and *Shigella* in freshly squeezed Orange juice, fresh oranges and wipping cloths collected from Public Markets and Street Booths in Guadalaraja, México: Incidence and Comparison of Analytical Routes. *Journal of Food Protection*, 69, 2595-2599.

Carinanos, M.C.C. (2005) Alteraciones y Riesgos Sanitários de Las Frutas e Hortalizas Frescas. *Alimentaria* , 361, 26-37.

Childs, N.M. and Poryzees, G.H. (1998). Food that help prevent disease: consumer attitudes and public policy implications. *British Food Journal*, 100, 419-426.

Cohen, N.; Hollingsworth, C.S.; Olson, R.B.; Laus, M.J. and Coli, W.M. (2005). Farm Food Safety Practices: a survey of New England Growers. *Food Protection Trends*, 25, 363-370.

Cox, L. J.; Keller, N.; Schothorst, M. (1998). The use and misuse of quantitative determinations of *Enterobacteriaceae* in food microbiology. *Journal of Applied Bacteriology*, Supplement, 65,. 237S-250S.

Croci, L.; Medici; D. de ; Scalfaro, C.; Foire, A. and Toti, L.(2002). The survival of hepatitis A virus in fresh produce. *International Journal of Food Microbiology*, 73, 29-34.

Cruz, A.G.da; Cenci, S.A. and Maia, M.C.A.(2006a). Quality assurance requiriments in produce processing. *Trends in Food Science and Technology*, 17, 406-411.

Cruz, A.G.da; Cenci, S.A. and Maia, M.C.A.(2006b). Requirements for HACCP system Implementation in a minimally processed plant . *Ciencia e Tecnologia de Alimentos*, 26, 404-409.

Cruz, A.G. da; Cenci, S.A. and Maia, M.C.A.(2006c). Good agricultural practices in a Brazilian produce plant. *Food Control*, 17, 781-788.

Daryani, A.; Ettehad, G.H.; Sharif, M.; Ghorbani, L. and Ziaei, H. (2008). Prevalence of intestinal parasites in vegetables consumed in Ardabil, Iran. *Food Control*, 19, 790-794.

De Roever, C. (1998). Microbiological safety evaluations and recommendations on fresh produce. *Food Control*, 9, 321-347.

Dewaal, C.S.; Hicks, G.; Barlow, K. Alderon, L. and Vegosen, L. (2006). Food Associated with Foodborne Illness Outbreaks from 1990 through 2003. *Food Protection Trends*, 26, 466-473.

Drofener, M.L.and Brinton, W.F. (1995). Survival of *E.Coli* and *Salmonella* populations in aerobic thermophilic composts as mesuared with DNA gene probes. *Zentralblatt fur Hygiene*, 197, p.387-397.

Early, R. (2005). Good agricultural practice and HACCP in fruit and vegetable cultivation. Improving the Safety of Fresh Fruit and Vegetables. In: Jongen, W. Improving the Safety of Fresh Fruit and Vegetables, 229-267. CRC Press: Boca Ranton

Erdogrul, O. and Sener, H. (2005). The *contamination of various fruit and vegetables with Enterobius vermicularis,* Ascaris eggs, *Entamoeba histolyca* and *Giardia* cysts. *Food Control*, 16, 559-562.

Fahrasmane, L.; Ganou, B and Aurore, G. (2007). Harmessing the health benefits of plant originating from the American Tropics in the diet. *Fruits*, 62, 213-222.

Fain, R. F. (1996). A Review of the Microbiological Safety of Fresh Salads. *Dairy Food and Environmental Sanitation*, 16,146-149.

Figueredo, R. M. (1999). SSOP- Padrões e Procedimentos Operacionais de Sanitizacão . São Paulo, Brazil: Câmara Brasileira do Livro.

Foster, J. W. and Hall, H. K. (1991). Inducible pH homeostasis and the acid tolerance response of *Salmonella typhimurium. Journal of Bacteriology*, 173, 5129-5135.

Frank, J. F.(2001). Microbial attachment to food and food contact surfaces. Advances in Food and Nutrition Research, 43, 320-380.

Froder, H.; Martins, C.G.; Souza, K.L. O de; Landgraf, M., Franco, B.D.G. and Destro M.T.(2007). Minimally processed vegetables salads: microbial quality evaluation. *Journal of Food Protection* , 5, 1277-1280.

Giese, J. H. (1991). Sanitatiion: The Key to Food Safety and Public Health. *Food Technology*, 45, 74-80.

Goodson, M. and Rowbury, R. J. (1989). Habituation to normally lethal acidity by prior growth of Escherichia coli at a sublethal acid pH value. *Letters in Applied Microbiology,* 8, 77-79.

Guam, T.G.; Blank, G.; Ismond, A. and Acker, R.V.(2005). Fate of foodborne pathogens in pesticide solutions. Journal of the Food Science and Agriculture, 81, 503-512.

Harris, L. J.; Farber, J. N.; Buechat, L. R.; Parish, M. E.; Suslow, T. V.; Garret, E. H. and Busta, F. F. Outbreaks associated with fresh produce: Incidence, growth, and survival of pathogens in fresh and fresh-cut produce. (2003). In: Institute of Food Technologists. Analysis and Evaluation of Preventive Control Measures for the Control and Reduction/Elimination of Microbial Hazards on Fresh and Fresh-Cut Produce. Avaiable in: <http://www.ift.org/cms/?pid=1000384>. Acessed: 16 may 2007

Howard, L.R.and Gonzalez, A.R. (2001). Food Safety and produce Operation: What is the future? *Hortscience*, 36, 33-39.

Hurst, W.C. (1995). Sanitation of Lightly Processed Fruits and Vegetables. *Hortscience*, 30, 22-24.

Institute of Food Technologists. Emerging microbiological food safety issues: Implications for control in the 21st. century. Chicago, 2000. Avaiable in: < http://www.ift.org/cms/?pid=1000377>. Acessed: 15 jun. 2004.

Inteak, A. (2004). Food Quality and Assurance: Principles and Practices. pp 140. CRC Press: Boca Ranton

International Commision on Microbiological Specifications for Foods. Microorganisms in foods 5: characteristics of microbial pathogens. Londres: Blackie Academic and Professional, 1996. 513 p.

International Fresh-Cut Produce Association. (1999). Food Safety Guidelines for the Fresh-Cut Produce Industry. 125 p.

Izumi, H.; Poubol, J.; Hisa, K. and Sera, K. (2008). Potential sources of microbial contamination of satsuma mandarin fruit in Japan, from production through packing shed. *Journal of Food Protection*, 71, 530-538

Jackson, C.; Archer, D.L.; Goodrich-Schineider, R.; Gravani, R.B.; Bihn, E.A. and Schneider, K.R. (2007). Determining the Effect of Good Agricultural Practices Awareness on Implementation: A multistate survey. *Food Protection Trends*, 27, 684-693.

Kato,M; Naka, K.; Yamamoto, H. and Kira, S.(2004).Assessing Education of FoodHandlers and Prerequisite Programs in Japanese HACCP Plants. *Food Protection Trends,* 24, 316-322.

Koneca-Matyjek, E.; Turlesjska, H.; Pelzner, U. and Szponar, L.(2005). Actual situation in the area of implementing quality assurance systems GMP,GHP and HACCP in Polish food production and Processing Plants. *Food Control*, 16, 1-9.

Kornacki, J.L. and Johnson. J.L. (2001). *Enterobacteriaceae*, coliforms, and *Escherichia coli* as quality and safety indicators. In: American Public Health Association Association. Compendium of Methods for the Microbiological Examination of Foods. 4 ed. Washington, D.C., 2001. p. 69-82.

Kokkinakis, K.; Boskou, G.; Fragkiadakis,G.A.; Kokkinaki, A. and Lapidakis, N.(2007). Microbiological quality of tomatoes and peppers produced under the good agricultural practices protocol AGRO 2-1 and 2-2 in Crete, Greece. *Food Control*, 18, 1538-1546..

Koopmans, M. and Duizer, E. (2004). Foodborne viruses: an emerging problem. *International Journal of Food Microbiology*, 90, 23- 41.

Kroll, R. G. and Patchet, R. A. (1992). Induced acid tolerance in *Listeria monocytogenes. Letters in Applied Microbiology*, 14, 224-227.

Leopolodo, O.R.; Iturriaga, M.H.; Tamplin, M.L.; Francisco, P.M.; Call, J.E.; Luchansky, J.B. and Escartin, E.F. (2008). Animal and Environmental Impact on the Presence and Distribution of *Salmonella* and *Escherichia coli* in Hydroponic Tomato Greenhouses. *Journal of Food Protection*, 71, 676-683.

Leong, Y-K; Xui, o-G and Chia, O-K.(2008). Survival of SA11 rotavirus in fresh fruit juices of pineapple, papya and honeydew melon. *Journal of Food Protection*, 71, 1035-1037.

Lesueur, C.; Gartner, M.; Knittl, P.; List, P.; Wimmer, S.; Sieler, V.; Fuerhacker, M. (2007). Pesticides residues in fruit and vegetable samples: analytical results of 2 year´s pesticide investigations. *Ernahrung*, 31, 247-259.

Lund, B. M. (1992). Ecosystems in vegetable foods. *Journal of Applied Bacteriology*, Symposium Supplement, 73, 115S-126S.

Madden, J.M.(1992). Microbial pathogens in fresh produce - the regulatory perspective. Journal of Food-Protection, 55, 821-823

Mendonca, A. Bacterial infiltration and internalization in fruits and vegetables. In: Produce Degration: Pathaways and Preventions. Taylor and Francis, 2005. Ch. 14, p. 441-462.

Mortimore, S. (2000). An example of some procedures used to assess HACCP systems within the food manufacturing industry. *Food Control*,11, 403-413.

Monge, R. and Chinchilla, M. (1996). Presence of Cryptosporidium oocysts in fresh vegetables. *Journal of Food Protection*, 59, 202-203.

Musgrove, C. (2008). Children's diet: looking the bigger picture. *International Food Information Service*, 40, p.4-6.

NACMF- National Advisory Committee on Microbiological Criteria for Foods. (1999). Microbiological safety evaluation and recommendations on fresh produce. *Food Control*, 10, 117-143.

Ness, A.R. and Powles, J.W. (1997). Fruit and Vegetables, and cardiovascular disease: a review. *International Journal of Epidemiology*, 26, p.1-13.

Nguyen-the, C. and Carlin, F. (1994). The microbiology of minimally processed fresh fruits and vegetables. Critical Review in Food Science and Nutrition, 34, 371-401.

O'Keeffe, M. and Kennedy, O. (1998). Residues: a food safety problem. *Journal of Food Safety*, 18, 297-319.

Olsen, A.R. and Zimmerman, M.L.(2003). Hard or Sharp Foreign Objects in Food. In: Hui, Y.H.; Bruinsma, B.; Gorham, J.R.; Nip, W.N.; Tong, P.S. and Ventresca, P. Food Plant Sanitation. pp.61-67. CRC Press: Boca Ranton

Orozco, R.L.; Iturriaga, M.H.; Tamplin, M.L.; Fratamico, P.M.; Call, J.E.; Luchansky, J.B. and Escartin, E.F. (2008). Animal and environmental impact on the presence and distribution of *Salmonella* and *Escherichia coli* in hydroponic tomato greenhouses. *Journal of Food Protection*, 71, 676-683 ;

Pabrua, F. P. (1996). Good Agricultural Practices: Methods to minimize microbial Risk. *Dairy, Food Environmental Sanitation*, 17, 523-526.

Paisley, J. and Skrzypczyk, S. (2005). Qualitative investigation of Differences in Benefits and challenges of eating Fruits vesus vegetables as perceived by Canadian women. *Journal of Nutrition Education Behaviour*, 37, 77-82.

Parish, M.E. (1997). Public Health and Nonpasteurized Juices. *Critical Reviews in Microbiology*, 23, 109-119.

Parish, M.E. (1998). Coliforms, Escherichia coli and Salmonella Serovars associated with a citrus-Processing faciltity implicated in a salmonellosis Outbreak. *Journal of Food Protection*, 61, 280-284.

Penteado, A.L. and Leitão, M.F.F.(2004a). Growth of *Salmonella Enteritidis* in melon, watermelon and papaya pulp stored at different times and temperatures. *Food Control*, 15, 369-373.

Penteado, A.L. and Leitão, M.F.F.(2004b). Growth of *Listeria monocytogenes* in melon, watermelon and papaya pulps. *International Journal of Food Microbiology*, 92, 89-94.

Pivarnik,D.; Donath, H.; Patnoad, M.S. and Roheim, C.(2005). New England Consumers′ Willingness to pay for Fresh Fruit and Vegetable Grown on Gap certified Farms. *Food Protection Trends*, 25, 256-266.

Pivarnik, L. F.; Richard, N.L.; Leydon, N. and Gable, R.K. (2006). New England Home Gardeners′ Food Safety Knowledge of Fresh Fruits and Vegetables. *Food Protection Trends*, 26, 298-309.

Porto, E. and Eiroa, M. N.U. (2001) . Ocurrence of Listeria monocytogenes in vegetables. *Dairy, Food And Environmental Sanitation*, 21, 12-16.

Poulsen, M.E. and Andersen, J.H. (2003). Results from monitoring of pesticides residues in fruit and vegetable on the Danish market. *Food Additives and Contaminants*, 20, 742-757.

Raspor, P. and Jevsnik, M. (2008). Good nutritional practice from producer to consumer.
Critical Reviews in Food Science and Nutrition, 48, 276-292 ;

Robertson, L.J. and Gjerde, B. (2001). Occurrence of parasites on fruits and vegetables in Norway. *Journal of Food Protection*, 64, 1793-1798

Rodrigues, N.R. (2006). Análise de Agrotóxicos: resíduos e monitoramento. *Multiciência*, 7, 1-8.

Ropkins, K. and Beck, A.J. (2003). Using HACPP to control organic chemical hazards in food wholesale, distribution, storage and retail. *Trends in Food Science and Technology*, 14, 374-389.

Roberto, C.D.; Brandão, S.C.B; Silva, C.A.B. da. (2005). Costs and investments of implementing and maintaining HACCP in a pasteurized milk plant. *Food Control*, 17, 599-603.

Saeed, T.; Sawaya, W.N.; Ahmad, N.; Rajagopal, S.; Al-Omair, A. and Al-Awadhi, F. (2001). Chlorinated pesticides residues in the total diet of Kuwait. *Food Control*, 12, 91-98.

Sapers, G.M. (2001). Efficacy of washing and sanitizing methods for disinfection of fresh fruit and vegetable products. *Food Technology and Biotechnology*, 39, 305-311.

Schuenzel, K. M. and Harrison, M. A. (2002). Microbial Antagonists of foodborne pathogens on fresh, minimally processed vegetables. *Journal of Food Protection*, 65, 1909-1915.

Seaton, L. (2001). Retailers assured by produce schemes. *Fresh Produce Journal*, Summer Supl.

Setiabuhdi, M., Theis, M. and Norback, J.(1998). Integrating Hazard Anaylisis and Critical point (HACCP) and sanitation for variable food safety. *Journal of the American Dietetic Association*, 98, 889-891

Sewell, A.M.and Farber, J.M. (2001). Foodborne outbreaks in Canada linked to produce. *Journal of Food Protection*, 64,1863-1877

Seymour, I.J. and Appleton, H. (2001). Foodborne viruses and fresh produce. *Journal of Applied Microbiology*, 91,. 759-773.

Silva, R S.R.P.; Verdin, S.E.F. and Pereira, D.C. (2007). Microbiological qualirty of minimally processed vegetables sold in Porto Alegre. *Brazilian Journal of Microbiology*, 38, 594-598.

Solomon E.B.; Potenski C.J. and Matthews K.R. (2002). Effect of Irrigation Method on transmission to and Persistence of *E. coli* 0157:H7. *Journal of Food Protection*, 65, 673-676.

Soriano, J.M.; Rico, H.; Molto, J.C. and Manes, J. (2002). Effect of introduction of HACCP on the microbiological quality of some restaurant meals. *Food Control*, 13, 253-261.

Sousa, W. (2001). Segurança Alimentar: Como conquistar o cliente pela confiança. *SuperHiper*, 9, 10-17.

Sperber, W.H. (2001). Hazard identification: from a quantitative to a qualitative approach. *Food Control*,12, 223-228

Sperber, W.H.; Stevenson, K.E.; Bernard, D.T.; Deibel, K.E.; Moberg, L.J.; Hontz, L.R. and Scott, V.N. (1998). The Role of Prerequisite Programs in Managing a HACCP system. *Dairy Food and Environmental Sanitation*, 18, 418-423.

Spurr, H. W. J. (1994). The microbial ecology of fruit and vegetable surface: Its relationship to postharvest biocontrol. In: Wilson, C. L. and WisniewskiI, M. E. Biological Control of Posthavervest Diseases: theory and practice. CRC Press: Boca Raton, 11-23.

Steele, M. and Odumeru, J. (2004). Irrigation Water as Source of Foodborne Pathogens Fruit and Vegetables. *Journal of Food Protection*, 67, 2839 – 2849.

Tomé M.M.; Vera, A.M. and Murcia, M.A. (2000). Improving the control of food production in catering establishments with particular reference to the safety of salads. *Food Control*, 11, 427- 445.

Tournas, V.M.(2005). Moulds and yeasts in fresh and minimally processed vegetables, and sprouts. *International Journal of Food Microbiology*, 90, 71-77.

Tumuhairwe, E.K.; Magel, R.; Madhusudan-Bhandary, N.C. and Khaitsa, M.L.(2008). Characterization of 386 non-typhoidal salmonellosis cases in North Dakota from 2000 to 2005. *Food-Protection-Trends*, 28, 304-313.

Untermann, F. (1998). Microbial Hazards in Food. *Food Control*, 9, 119-126.

Vanetti, M. C. D. (2004). Segurança microbiológica em produtos minimamente processados. In: Encontro Nacional sobre Processamento Mínimo de Frutas e Hortaliças, 3, 2004, Viçosa. Resumos. p.30-32.

Vojdani, J.D.; Beuchat, L.R. and Tauxe, R.V. (2008). Juice-associated Outbreaks of Human Illness in the United States, 1995 through 2005. *Journal of Food Protection*, 71, 356-364.

Wallace, C. and Williams, T.(2001). Prerequisites: a help or a hindrance to HACCP. *Food Control,* 12, 235-240.

Wells, J. M. and Butterfield, J. E. (1997). *Salmonella* contamination associated with bacterial soft rot of fresh fruits and vegetables in the marketplace. *Plant Disease*, 81, 867-872.

Wiley, R.C.(1994). Minimally Processed Refrigerated Fruits and Vegetables. pp 368. Chapman and Hall: New York.

Williamson, G. (1996). Protective Effects of fruits and Vegetables in the diet. *Nutrition and Food Science* , 96, p.6-10.

Willock, F., Tobback, P. and Henrickx, M. (1994). Microbial Safety Assurance of minimally processed vegetables by implementation of the Hazards Analysis Critical Control Points. *Acta Alimentaria*, 23, 221-238.

Winter, C.K.(2000).Pesticides Residues in Food Supply. In: Helferich,W. and Winter, C.K. Food Toxicology ; pp. 163- 185. CRC Press: Boca Raton.

Winter, C.K.(2005). Pesticides Residues in Fruits and Vegetables. In: Jongen, W. Improving the Safety of Fresh Fruit and Vegetables; 135-155. CRC Press: Boca Raton.

Wright, J. R.; Summer, S.S.; Hackney, C.R.; Pierson, M.D. and Zoecklein, B.W. (2000). A survey of Virginia Apple Producers' Practices. *Dairy, Food and Environmental Sanitation*, 20, 190-195.

In: Fruit and Vegetable Consumption and Health
Editors: Anton Papareschi and Harvey Eppolito
ISBN: 978-1-60741-596-1

Chapter II

Dietary Intake Of Potentially Toxic Elements From Vegetables

***M. Azizur Rahman*[a], *M. Mahfuzur Rahman*[b], *Ismail M. M. Rahman*[c] and *H. Hasegawa*[d]**

[a]Graduate School of Natural Science and Technology,
Kanazawa University, Kakuma, Japan
[b]Department of Botany, Jahangirnagar Univeristy, Savar, Bangladesh
[c]Graduate School of Natural Science and Technology,
Kanazawa University, Kakuma, Japan
Department of Chemistry, University of Chittagong, Chittagong 4331, Bangladesh
[d]Graduate School of Natural Science and Technology,
Kanazawa University, Kakuma, Japan

Abstract

Toxic elements e.g., arsenic (As), cadmium (Cd), chromium (Cr), copper (Cu), lead (Pb), and zinc (Zn) are the chief environmental pollutants which can cause deleterious health effects in humans. Inhalation and consumption of metal-contaminated food are the major pathways of metal entrance into human body. Cultivation of crop plants in the metal-contaminated soils induces the bioaccumulation of toxic elements in the food chain. Among different food items, vegetables have major contribution in the daily diet, and the heavy metal contamination of vegetables poses a threat to human health with the prevalence of skin and gastrointerestinal cancer.

The uptake and bioaccumulation of toxic elements in vegetables are influenced by a number of factors such as atmospheric deposition, metal concentrations in soil, soil characteristics, and duration of cultivation. Cultivation areas near highways are exposed to atmospheric pollution in the form of metal containing aerosols which can be deposited on leaves of vegetables and then absorbed. The magnitude of heavy metal deposition on vegetable surfaces varied with morpho-physiological nature of the vegetables. Post-harvest activities, such as transportation, marketing, cooking, etc., may also influence the deposition of toxic elements in vegetables. Incorporation of toxic elements during transportation and marketing of vegetable can be occurred due to the use of contaminated water. Higher heavy metal content in vegetables from urban area then those from rural areas may be due to the contribution of urban activities which elevates heavy metal loads in atmospheric deposition and consequently in the edible part of the vegetables. Cooking has definite influence to the content of toxic elements in cooked items if the heavy metal concentrations in the cooking water are high.

Vegetable consumption varies with age group, food habit, as well as vegetable availability. For example the mean daily vegetable consumption among the European people is 153 g (ranged between 109-241 g) while it is around 250g among the South Asian people. Vegetables occupy a substantial proportion of the daily diet for the South-East Asian people, especially the Japanese, Korean and Chinese people. Thus, whatever the metal contents in vegetables are, their intake in human is, off course, dependent on the total vegetable consumption. In this review, the contribution of vegetables in dietary intake of toxic elements has been discussed from a common platform.

Introduction

Metals comprise about 75% of the known elements and have been used from the beginning of ancient human civilization. Since the beginning of the Industrial Age, metals have been emitted to and deposited in the environment [1]. In some cases, metals have accumulated in terrestrial and aquatic environments in high concentrations and cause harm to animals and humans via ingestion of soil and/or dust, food, and water; inhalation of polluted air; and absorption via the skin from polluted soils, water and air [2]. Increasing use of metals with the boom of population and economy, especially in the developing countries, could contaminate the soil and water causing the deterioration of environmental quality and posing threat to human health. [1].

Metals can be classified in to light, heavy, semimetal (i.e. metalloids), toxic, and trace, depending on several physico-chemical characteristics [3]. Certain metals and metalloids, commonly known as micronutrients, are essential for plant growth and animal health. Micronutrients include B, Cu, Fe, Zn, Mn, Mo. In addition, As, Co, Cr, Ni, Se, Sn, and V are especially essential in animal nutrition. Micronutrients are also known as "trace elements" since they are needed in only small quantities. In excess, trace elements can be toxic to living beings though their deficiency is also a problem to the normal growth of plant, microbes, and animals [1]. Important trace elements in the environment are As, Ag, B, Ba, Be, Cd, Co, Cr, Cu, Hg, Mn, Mo, Ni, Pb, Se, and Zn. However, the trace elements are also essential for organisms at low concentrations in most of the cases [4].

The trace elements can be derived from both natural and anthropogenic sources. Natural (geogenic) sources includes parent rocks and metallic minerals, and the anthropogenic sources include agriculture (fertilizers, pesticides, herbicides, and animal manures), mining, smelting, and sewage sludge and scrap disposal [4]. Anthropogenic deposition is a major mechanism for heavy metal input in the environment. Soil is the major recipient of trace elements in terrestrial environment, while sediments are the major sink in aquatic environment. Leaching of heavy metals or transport via mobile colloids can contaminate groundwater. On the other hand, runoff and drainage of the heavy metals via sediments can contaminate freshwater environment [2, 4].

Bioaccumulation of toxic elements in the food chain can be especially dangerous to human health. The toxic metals can enter into the human body by either inhalation or by ingestion; and ingestion is the main route of exposure to these elements [5]. For most of the people the main route of exposure to trace elements is diet except occupational exposures at related industries [6]. The exposure of heavy metal through the food chain has been reported in many countries, particularly in developing countries, and received huge attention from the governmental and non-governmental agencies [7-10]. The concern by environmentalists of the accumulation of toxic metals in the food chain, and the harmful effects on the environment by those metals has escalated in recent years. Once these metals enter into the biological systems they disturb the normal biochemical processes, and in some cases it can be fatal [11]. Regulations have been set up for the industries and other structures that discharging pollutants into the environment in many countries to control the emission of trace elements and their subsequent health effects.

Vegetables constitute essential components of the diet, by contributing proteins, vitamins, iron, calcium, and other nutrients. A constant supply of essential bioavailable trace elements is necessary and highly recommended for daily life [12]. Vegetables also act as buffering agents for acid substances obtained during the digestion process and contain both essential and toxic elements over a wide range of concentrations [13]. Vegetable is one of the major diets for the populations of many countries. A Bangladeshi individual, regardless of gender, consumes an average of 130 g vegetables per day (leafy and non-leafy) and in the total diet, the proportion varied from 12 - 21% [14, 15]. However, the recommended requirement of vegetables in daily diets is 200 g $person^{-1}$ day^{-1} [16]. The Japanese diet is substantially high in vegetables, fish and soy products, and low in saturated fats and sugar [17]. A large proportion of the adult United States population eats no vegetables (0.17) or fruit (0.41) on any given day [18]. Based on a comprehensive literature review, the National Academy of Sciences (NAS) concluded that diet influences the risk of several major chronic diseases and recommended eating five or more daily servings of a combination of vegetables and fruit, especially green and yellow vegetables and citrus fruit [19]. The US Department of Agriculture (USDA) and the Department of Health and Human Services (DHHS) recommend as part of their food guidance system that the daily diet include two to three servings of fruit and three to five servings of vegetables [20, 21]. But about 45 percent of the population had no servings of fruit or juice and 22 percent had no servings of a vegetable on the recall day. Only 27 percent consumed the three or more servings of vegetables and 29 percent had the two or more servings of fruit recommended by the US Departments of Agriculture and of Health and Human Services; 9 percent had both [22]. The people of Mediterranean countries consume about 248 g (113-456 g) of vegetables a day [23]. On the other hand, vegetable is neglected in the daily diet of Arabian countries.

Recently, vegetable becomes popular in daily diet of health conscious people because of its antioxidant properties. A wide number of vegetables are consumed by the population of different countries worldwide. Heavy metal uptake in vegetables and other food crops due to soil, water, and atmospheric contamination is a great threat to the food quality and food safety [5]. The uptake and bioaccumulation of trace elements in vegetables are influenced by a number of factors such as climate, atmospheric depositions, the concentrations of trace elements in the soils, the nature of soils on which the vegetables are grown, and the exposure time [24, 25]. Trace elements from air may also be deposited on vegetables during post-harvest activities such as transportation, marketing, etc. [6]. Vegetables accumulate trace elements from contaminated soils and store them in their edible and inedible parts with various concentrations, as well as from deposits on parts of vegetables exposed to the air from polluted environment [26].

Dietary intake of trace elements from vegetables is an important concern because of their potential health risks, and detrimental effects on the environment. It has been reported that nearly half of the mean ingestion of lead, cadmium, and mercury through food is of plant origin (fruits, vegetables, and cereals) [5]. Previously, a large scale study on trace elements in vegetables and fruits from the Valparaiso region of Chile has been conducted by Pinochet et al. [27]. Trace elements in various common vegetables collected from two typical growing areas of northwestern Greece were studied by Stalikas et al. [28]. Ursinyova et al. [29] reported the contents of cadmium, lead, and mercury in crops, vegetables from selected regions of Slovakia and compared to the provisional tolerable weekly intake as recommended by the world health organization (WHO) [30]. The cadmium and lead were determined in lettuce, potato, soy beans, and wheat in the United States [31, 32]. The trace elements in some vegetables, fruits, and cereals in Egypt were also reported in literatures [33]. The trace elements in vegetables grown in the greater industrial areas of North Greece (Thessaloniki) was investigated too and elevated concentrations, in some cases exceeding the maximum permissible limit of human consumption, was observed, particularly for Pb, Cd, Zn and As [25, 34]. In this review, the contribution of vegetables in dietary intake of some important trace elements such as arsenic (As), cadmium (Cd), chromium (Cr), copper (Cu), lead (Pb), and zinc (Zn), and their effects to human health has been discussed for different countries as reported in literatures.

Dietary Intake Of Toxic Elements From Vegetables

Arsenic (As)

Sources of human exposure:

Arsenic is a naturally occurring element that is widely distributed in the Earth's crust. Arsenic is classified chemically as a metalloid, having both properties of a metal and a nonmetal; however, it is frequently referred to as a metal [35]. However, arsenic is usually found in the environment combined with other elements such as oxygen, chlorine, and sulfur. Arsenic combined with these elements is called inorganic arsenic. Arsenic combined with carbon and hydrogen is referred to as organic arsenic. Arsenic occurs naturally in soil and minerals and it therefore may enter the air, water, and land from wind-blown dust and may get into water from runoff and leaching. Volcanic eruptions are another source of arsenic.

Table 1: Arsenic content in common vegetables collected from arsenic-prone villages of Bangladesh (Personal communication).

Vegetables (Scientific Name)	Arsenic Content (mg kg^{-1} Fresh Weight)
Bean (*Lablab niger*)	0.44±0.02 - 0.40±0.21
Bitter gourd (*Momordica charantia*)	0.37±0.05
Bottle gourd (*Lagenaria siceraria*)	BDL
Brinjal (*Solanum melongena*)	0.24±0.01 - 0.26±0.07
Chilli (*Capsicum frutescens*)	0 - 0.87±0.48
Green papaya (*Carica papaya*)	0.08±0.03
Mint (*Mentha viridis*)	0.59±0.07 - 0.56±0.04
Okra (*Abelmoschus esculentus*)	BDL
Palwal (*Trichosanthes dioica*)	BDL
Potato (*Solanum tuberosum*)	0.12±0.07
Pumpkin leaf (*Cucurbita maxima*)	0.41±0.07
Red amaranth (*Amaranthus gangeticus*)	0.16±0.03
String bean (*Vigna sesquipedalis*)	1.26±0.06 - 0.88±0.04
Sweet gourd (pumpkin) (*Cucurbita maxima*)	0.11±0.01 - 0.12±0.02
Tomato (*Lycopersicon esculentum*)	0.08±0.01 - 0.54±0.31

Data are presented as mean ± SD ($n = 3$). 'BDL' = below detection limit.

Arsenic is associated with ores containing metals, such as copper and lead. Arsenic may enter the environment during the mining and smelting of these ores. Small amounts of arsenic also may be released into the atmosphere from coal-fired power plants and incinerators because coal and waste products often contain some arsenic [35].

Many common arsenic compounds can dissolve in water. Thus, arsenic can get into lakes, rivers, or underground water by dissolving in rain or snow or through the discharge of industrial wastes. Some of the arsenic will stick to particles in the water or sediment on the bottom of lakes or rivers, and some will be carried along by the water. Ultimately, most arsenic ends up in the soil or sediment.

Health effects:

Inorganic arsenic has been recognized as a human poison since ancient times. Perhaps the single-most characteristic effect of long-term oral exposure to inorganic arsenic is a pattern of skin changes. These include patches of darkened skin and the appearance of small "corns" or "warts" on the palms, soles, and torso, and are often associated with changes in the blood vessels of the skin. Skin cancer may also develop. Swallowing arsenic has also been reported to increase the risk of cancer in the liver, bladder, and lungs. The Department of Health and Human Services (DHHS) has determined that inorganic arsenic is known to be a human carcinogen (a chemical that causes cancer). The International Agency for Research on Cancer (IARC) has determined that inorganic arsenic is carcinogenic to humans. EPA also has classified inorganic arsenic as a known human carcinogen [35]. Chronic arsenic poisoning associated with groundwater contamination has been reported in many countries, often where poor nutritional status is concomitantly found, and it has been suggested that the poor nutritional status affects the toxicity and metabolism of arsenic [36-41]. A case-control study conducted in Bangladesh showed that malnourished individuals are more often found among patients with arsenicosis than among the non-exposed population [42].

Dietary intake:

As reported in the literatures, the total arsenic contents in vegetable products were < 0.004 to 0.303 mg kg^{-1} fresh weight [43-46], which is within the range of values found in the samples of Bangladesh (Table 1). The average arsenic concentration in the vegetables collected from some arsenic prone areas of Bangladesh was 0.28 mg kg^{-1} fresh weight (ranging between 0.25 and 0.38 mg kg^{-1} fresh weight), which was higher than that of the United Kingdom, 0.003 mg kg^{-1} fresh weight [47], and Croatia, 0.0004 mg kg^{-1} fresh weight [48]. However, string beans collected from Bangladesh were found to have highest mean arsenic content (between 0.88±0.04 and 1.26±0.06 mg kg^{-1} fresh weight). Arsenic content in vegetables of some other countries have also been reported in literatures. Voutsa et al. [25] investigated the arsenic content in vegetables of Greece and found the lowest in *Daucas carota* L. (Carrots) (0.02-0.05 mg kg^{-1} dry weight) while the highest in *Cichorium endivia* (Endive) (0.13-0.19 mg kg^{-1} dry weight) (Table 3).

A Bangladeshi individual, regardless of gender, consumes an average of 130 – 200 g of vegetables per day (leafy and non-leafy) [14, 15]. Thus, the average dietary intake of total arsenic from vegetables by the inhabitants of arsenic prone area in Bangladesh was estimated to be 0.015 – 0.161 mg day^{-1}. In another study Rahman et al. [49] reported that the average dietary intake of arsenic from vegetables by the inhabitants of Bangladesh was 0.0147 mg day^{-1}.

However, the recommended daily dietary intake of vegetables is 200 g $person^{-1}$ day^{-1}, though the availability of vegetables is only about $1/5^{th}$ of the suggested requisite in Bangladesh [15]. If we consider that every person is able to fulfill the recommended amount of vegetables in their daily diets, the estimated average daily dietary intake of arsenic from vegetables in Bangladesh would be 0.0758 mg day^{-1}. The average intake of total arsenic from vegetable by an adult has been reported as 0.012 mg day^{-1} in Belgium [50], 0.015 mg day^{-1} in Netherlands [51], 0.0592 mg day^{-1} in Canada [43], 0.060 mg day^{-1} in Sweden [52], 0.160–0.280 mg day^{-1} in Japan [53], and 0.291 mg day^{-1} in Spain [45]. Per capita vegetable consumption by a Greek adult is reported to be about 240 g (the mean total daily availability of main foods, except water and beverages, per capita in Greece is 1575 g in which vegetables represent 15.3% of the total daily diet) [54]. On the basis of this calculation diet, daily dietary intake of arsenic via fresh vegetables in Greece has been reported as 0.02-0.63 μg day^{-1} from cabbage, 0.01-0.04 μg day^{-1} from carrot, 0.004-0.06 μg day^{-1} from leek, 0.04-0.26 μg day^{-1} from lettuce, 0.31-0.46 μg day^{-1} from Endive. If the mean daily consumption availability of these five vegetables was 61 g (as reported in literature), a total of 0.38-1.5 μg of As would be taken day^{-1} by a Greek adult. Moreover, assuming the similar content of arsenic in most vegetables in the Greek diet and considering the mean daily vegetable consumption availability as 241 g (as reported in literature), the total daily intake of arsenic would be 1.5-5.9 μg [54]. Thus, the total dietary intake of arsenic via vegetables in Greece was calculated to be 1.7% of the provisional tolerable daily intake (PTDI) according to the WHO [30, 55].

As found in the literature, the inorganic arsenic species content in diets ranges between 40% [56], 65% [43], 95-96% [57] and 100% [58]. Based on those reports, we can assume that at least 50% of the total arsenic in the vegetable samples is inorganic. Therefore, the daily dietary intake of inorganic arsenic from vegetables in Chittagong areas of Bangladesh would be at least 0.288 mg to 0.047 mg. From a toxicological point of view, inorganic arsenic compounds are the most toxic, and according to the WHO [59], a daily intake of 2 μg of inorganic arsenic per kg body weight should not be exceeded to minimize the health risk.

Cadmium (Cd)

Sources of human exposure:

Cadmium is one of six substances banned by the European Union's Restriction on Hazardous Substances (RoHS) directive, which bans certain hazardous substances in electronics [60]. Cadmium is also a potential environmental hazard. Human exposures to environmental cadmium are primarily the result of the burning of fossil fuels and municipal wastes [61], and the production of nickel-cadmium batteries, pigments, plastics, and other synthetics. Cadmium occurs in the earth's crust at a concentration of 0.1–0.5 mg kg^{-1} and is commonly associated with zinc, lead, and copper ores. It is also a natural constituent of ocean water with average levels between <5 and 110 ng L^{-1}. The cadmium concentration of natural surface water and groundwater is usually <1 μg L^{-1} [62]. Non-ferrous metal mining and refining, manufacture and application of phosphate fertilizers, fossil fuel combustion, and waste incineration and disposal are the main anthropogenic sources of cadmium in the environment. Water sources near cadmium-emitting industries, both with historic and current operations; have shown a marked elevation of cadmium in water sediments and aquatic organisms. Concentrations of cadmium in these polluted waters have ranged from <1.0 to 77 μg L^{-1}. Cadmium from polluted soil and water can accumulate in plants and organisms, thus entering the food supply [62].

Smoking greatly increases exposure to cadmium, as tobacco leaves naturally accumulate high amounts of cadmium. It has been estimated that tobacco smokers are exposed to 1.7 μg cadmium per cigarette, and about 10% is inhaled when smoked. A geometric mean blood cadmium level for a heavy smoker has been reported as high as 1.58 μg L^{-1}, compared to the estimated national mean of 0.47 μg L^{-1} for all adults [62]. The largest source of cadmium exposure for nonsmoking adults and children is through dietary intake. The estimated daily intakes of cadmium in nonsmoking adult males and females living in the United States are 0.35 and 0.30 μg Cd kg^{-1} day^{-1}, respectively. In general, leafy vegetables such as lettuce and spinach and staples such as potatoes and grains contain relatively high values of cadmium [62]. Peanuts, soybeans, and sunflower seeds have naturally high levels of cadmium.

Health effects:

The primary route of exposure in industrial settings is inhalation [63]. Current research has found that cadmium toxicity may be carried into the body by zinc binding proteins; in particular, proteins that contain zinc finger protein structures. Zinc and cadmium are in the same group on the periodic table, contain the same common oxidation state (+2), and when ionized are almost the same size. Due to these similarities, cadmium can replace zinc in many biological systems, in particular, systems that contain softer ligands such as sulfur. Cadmium can bind up to ten times more strongly than zinc in certain biological systems, and is notoriously difficult to remove. In addition, cadmium can replace magnesium and calcium in certain biological systems, although these replacements are rare [64].

However, there have been notable instances of toxicity as the result of long-term exposure to cadmium in contaminated food and water. In the decades following World War II, Japanese mining operations contaminated the Jinzu River with cadmium and traces of other toxic metals. As a consequence, cadmium accumulated in the rice crops growing along the riverbanks downstream of the mines. The local agricultural communities consuming the contaminated rice developed Itai-itai disease and renal abnormalities, including proteinuria and glucosuria [65].

Acute inhalation exposure to high levels of cadmium in humans may result in effects on the lung, such as bronchial and pulmonary irritation. A single acute exposure to high levels of cadmium can result in long-lasting impairment of lung function [61, 62]. Chronic inhalation and oral exposure of humans to cadmium results in a build-up of cadmium in the kidneys that can cause kidney disease, including proteinuria, a decrease in glomerular filtration rate, and an increased frequency of kidney stone formation [61]. Other effects noted in occupational settings from chronic exposure of humans to cadmium in air are effects on the lung, including bronchiolitis and emphysema.

Dietary intake:

Cadmium content has been reported in various common vegetables of many countries. In a study Bahemuka and Mubofu [13] reported that the cadmium content in vegetables of Tanzania ranged between 0.1 and 0.6 mg kg^{-1} dry weight. The highest content of cadmium was in African spinach (*Spinacia oleracea* L.) (0.3-0.6 mg kg^{-1} dry weight) while the lowest was in Leafy cabbages (*Brassica oleracea var. capitata* L.), about 0.1 mg kg^{-1} dry weight) (Table 4). Cadmium contents have also been reported in vegetables of Saudi Arabia (the lowest in Cucumber (*Cucumis sativa* L.) and Cabbage (*Brassica oleracea* var. *capitata* L.), about 0.59 mg kg^{-1} dry weight and the highest in Watercress (*Nasturtium officinale*, *N. microphyllum*), about 1.22 mg kg^{-1} dry weight) (Table 2) [12]; Greece (the lowest in Carrots (*Daucas carota* L.), about 0.17-0.41 mg kg^{-1} dry weight and the highest in Cabbages (*Brassica oleracea* L.), about 0.26-1.03 mg kg^{-1} dry weight) (Table 3) [25, 54]; India (the lowest in Chinese onion (*Allium cepa* L.), about 5.7-25.0 mg kg^{-1} dry weight and the highest in Spinach (*Spinacia oleracea* L.), about 6.5-32.0 mg kg^{-1} dry weight) (Table 5) [66].

The above data reveal that cadmium content in same vegetable differs from country to country. According to above reports, cadmium content in vegetables of India is many folds higher than those of other countries. It might be because the metal uptake in vegetables is influenced by several factors such as metal concentrations in agricultural soils, soil pH, physico-chemical characteristics of the soil, soil classification, etc. Moreover, vegetable consumption (per person per day) is not same for the residents of different regions. It was reported that the average consumption of leafy vegetables is 108 g per person per day in the coastal region of Tanzania [13] while it is 130-200 g per person per day in rural Bangladesh [14, 15]. Thus, dietary intake of cadmium would very from region to region. It was estimated

Table 2: Heavy metal concentrations in some common vegetables of Saudi Arabia [12].

Vegetables (Scientific Name)	Heavy metal contents (mg kg^{-1})			
	Cd	Cu	Pb	Zn
Cucumber (*Cucumis sativa* L.)	0.59	2.48	4.26	32.30
Egg-plant (*Solanum melongena* L.)	0.69	2.93	4.57	50.70
Carrots (*Daucas carota* L.)	0.81	0.98	7.94	9.60
Lettuce (*Lactuca sativa)*	1.04	0.90	3.70	42.00
Spinach (*Spinacia oleracea* L.)	0.77	2.71	9.44	9.60
Green pepper (*Capsicum frutescens)*	0.80	4.49	1.90	8.51
Onion (*Allium cepa* L.)	0.76	1.07	10.29	17.60
Watercress (*Nasturtium microphyllum)*	1.22	1.96	14.37	105.20
Cabbages *Brassica oleracea* L.)	0.59	0.43	-	14.90
Potatoes (*Solanum tuberosum* L.)	0.84	0.88	2.81	4.5
Tomato (*Lycopersicon esculentum* L.)	0.77	4.47	2.59	14.40

that if the mean content of cadmium in vegetables of Tanzania was 0.20 mg kg^{-1} and if the average vegetable consumption was 108 g per person per day, the contribution of green vegetable to daily dietary intake of cadmium would be 0.02 mg. In contrast, if the vegetable consumption is 130-200 g per person per day by the Indian people (as a neighboring country of Bangladesh, the food habit and food consumption of the Indian people is almost same), the estimated contribution of vegetables to daily dietary intake would be 0.74-5.00 mg. Voutsa and Samara [54] reported dietary intake of Cd from five vegetable species from Greece as 0.4-1.8 μg day^{-1} from cabbage, 0.2-0.3 μg day^{-1} from carrot, 0.1-0.2 μg day^{-1} from leek, 0.4-0.6 μg day^{-1} from lettuce, 1.1-1.7 μg day^{-1} from Endive, with a total of 2.2-4.6 μg day^{-1} (if the mean daily consumption availability of five listed vegetables is considered to be 61 g as reported in literature). Assuming the similar content of cadmium in most vegetables in the Greek diet and considering the mean daily vegetable consumption availability as 241 g (as reported in literature) [55], the total daily intake of cadmium would be 8.7-18 μg which represents 15.7% of the provisional tolerable daily intake (PTDI) according to the WHO [30, 55]. Other estimates made from various countries have shown that the daily dietary intake of cadmium from vegetables is between 10-20 mg [67].

Chromium (Cr)

Sources of human exposure:

Chromium (Cr) is the seventh most abundant element on earth crust [68]. Due to its wide industrial use, chromium is considered a serious environmental pollutant. Chromium is found in all phases of the environment, including air, water and soil. Human can be exposed to chromium by breathing air, drinking water, or eating food containing chromium or through skin contact with chromium or chromium compounds. The level of chromium in air and water is generally low. The concentration of total chromium in air (both Cr(III) and Cr(VI)) generally ranges between 0.01 and 0.03 μg m^{-3}. Chromium concentrations in drinking water (mostly as Cr(III)) are generally very low, less than 2 μg l^{-1}. For the general population, eating foods that contain chromium is the most likely route of Cr(III) exposure. Cr(III) occurs naturally in many fresh vegetables, fruits, meat, yeast, and grain [69].

Chromium compounds are highly toxic to plants and are detrimental to their growth and development [70]. Although some crops are not affected by low Cr concentration (3.8×10^{-4} μM) [71, 72], Cr is toxic to most higher plants at 100 μM kg^{-1} dry weight [73, 74]. Contamination of soil and ground water due to the use of chromium in various anthropomorphic activities has become a serious source of concern to plant and animal scientists over the past decade. The stable forms of chromium are the trivalent Cr(III) and the hexavalent Cr(VI) species, although there are various other valence states which are unstable and short-lived in biological systems [75].

Health effects:

Chromium can be both beneficial and toxic to animals and humans depending on its oxidations state and concentration. At low concentration, Cr(III) is essential for animal and human health that helps the body use sugar, protein, and fat [68]. In general, Cr(VI) is absorbed by the body more easily than Cr(III), but once inside the body, Cr(VI) is changed to Cr(III). Although Cr(III) in small amounts is a nutrient needed by the body, swallowing large amounts of Cr(III) may cause health problems [69]. An intake of 50–200 μg of Cr(III) per day is recommended for adults. Without chromium(III) in the diet, the body loses its ability to use sugars, proteins, and fat properly, which may result in weight loss or decreased growth, improper function of the nervous system, and a diabetic-like condition [69].

Chromium(VI) is considered the most toxic form of chromium which usually occurs in association with oxygen as chromate (CrO_4^{2-}) or dichromate ($Cr_2O_7^{2-}$) oxyanions. Chromium(III) is less mobile, less toxic, and is mainly found bound to organic matter in soil and aquatic environments [70]. The health effects resulting from exposure to Cr(III) and Cr(VI) are fairly well described in the literature. Chromium(VI) is believed to be primarily responsible for the increased lung cancer rates observed in workers who were exposed to high levels. The EPA has determined that Cr(VI) in air is a human carcinogen. The EPA has also determined that there is insufficient information to determine whether Cr(VI) in water or food and Cr(III) are human carcinogens [69].

Dietary intake:

However, chromium content in leafy vegetables has been reported in many countries. In a study Voutsa et al. [25] reported 0.08-9.72 mg kg^{-1} dry weight of Cr in different vegetables of Greece (Table 3). Voutsa et al. [25] found 0.86-9.72 mg kg^{-1} dry weight of Cr in Lettuce (*Lactuca sativa*) while its content was about 0.13-3.42 mg kg^{-1} dry weight in Leek (*Allium ampeloprasum* var. *porrum* L.) (Table 3). Chromium in vegetables of India has also been reported by Gupta et al. [66]. The content of Cr in Indian vegetables ranged between 40.3-115.4 mg kg^{-1} dry weight (Table 5). The highest Cr content was found in Spinach (*Spinacia oleracea* L.), about 74.0-115.4 mg kg^{-1} dry weight and the lowest was found in Chinese onion (*Allium cepa* L.), about 40.3-53.2 mg kg^{-1} dry weight. Cr content in Pakistani vegetables ranged between 0.1±0.00 mg kg^{-1} dry weight (in Mustard (*Brassica juncea*)) and 1.2±0.01 mg kg^{-1} dry weight (in Coriander (*Coriandrum sativum*)) (Table 6) [76].

Table 2: Heavy metal concentrations in some common vegetables of Saudi Arabia [12].

Vegetables (Scientific Name)	Heavy metal contents (mg kg^{-1})			
	Cd	Cu	Pb	Zn
Cucumber (*Cucumis sativa* L.)	0.59	2.48	4.26	32.30
Egg-plant (*Solanum melongena* L.)	0.69	2.93	4.57	50.70
Carrots (*Daucas carota* L.)	0.81	0.98	7.94	9.60
Lettuce (*Lactuca sativa*)	1.04	0.90	3.70	42.00
Spinach (*Spinacia oleracea* L.)	0.77	2.71	9.44	9.60
Green pepper (*Capsicum frutescens*)	0.80	4.49	1.90	8.51
Onion (*Allium cepa* L.)	0.76	1.07	10.29	17.60
Watercress (*Nasturtium microphyllum*)	1.22	1.96	14.37	105.20
Cabbages *Brassica oleracea* L.)	0.59	0.43	-	14.90
Potatoes (*Solanum tuberosum* L.)	0.84	0.88	2.81	4.5
Tomato (*Lycopersicon esculentum* L.)	0.77	4.47	2.59	14.40

Chromium is usually found in its trivalent form in biological and food samples [77] while the hexavalent form is the most toxic. The average dietary intake of chromium as estimated by Biego et al. [78] was 98 µg day^{-1}, which is between those recommended by the United States (50-100 µg day^{-1}) [79]. Anderson et al. [80] reported that chromium contents of grain products, fruits, and vegetables vary widely, with some foods providing >20 g/serving. Van Cauwenbergh et al. [81] reported that the mean Cr intake Belgium was 53±31 µg day^{-1}, which is similar to levels found for most other countries and is situated at the lower end of the recommended range for a safe and adequate daily dietary intake. The mean total daily availability of main foods, except water and beverages, per capita in Greece is 1575 g in which vegetables represent 15.3% of the total daily diet [54]. Daily dietary intake of chromium via fresh vegetables in Greece has been reported as 0.3-13 µg day^{-1} from cabbage, 0.06-6 µg day^{-1} from carrot, 0.05-1.4 µg day^{-1} from leek, 0.6-8.7 µg day^{-1} from lettuce, 1.2-13 µg day^{-1} from Endive, with a total of 2.2-42.0 µg day^{-1} from these five vegetables (if the mean daily consumption availability of the five vegetables was considered to be 61 g, as reported literature [54]). Assuming the similar content of chromium in most vegetables in the Greek diet and considering the mean daily vegetable consumption availability as 241 g (as reported in literature [55]), the total daily intake of Cr would be 8.7-166 µg.

Copper (Cu)

Sources of human exposure:

Copper is among the major toxic elements contaminants in the environment with various anthropogenic and natural sources. A range of Cu based products have been historically and are currently used as fungicides [82]. Copper may also deposit in agricultural soils from wastewater, mine, and industrial discharges. Although it is an essential micronutrient for normal plant metabolism, playing an important role in a large number of metalloenzymes, photosynthesis-related plastocyanin, and membrane structure, copper has been reported to be among the most toxic of toxic elementss [83, 84]. People may be exposed to copper by breathing air, drinking water, eating food, and by skin contact with soil, water and other copper-containing substances [85].

Health effects:

Copper is an essential mineral for human health and at the same time can be toxic, depending upon the amounts ingested. However, exposure to higher doses can be harmful. Long term exposure to copper dust can irritate your nose, mouth, and eyes, and cause headaches, dizziness, nausea, and diarrhea. Intentionally high intakes of copper can cause liver and kidney damage and even death. We do not know if copper can cause cancer in humans. EPA does not classify copper as a human carcinogen because there are no adequate human or animal cancer studies [85]. There are numerous reports of acute gastrointestinal effects in humans after ingestion of large amounts of copper in drinking water or beverages. The most prevalent effects are nausea and vomiting, which typically occur shortly after ingestion and are not persistent [86-90].

Copper is associated with bone health, immune function and increased frequency of infections, cardiovascular risk and alterations in cholesterol metabolism. Its metabolism is tightly intertwined with other microminerals and its deficiency is known to impair iron mobilisation, resulting in secondary iron deficiency [91].

Dietary intake:

Copper uptake by vegetable plants from soils and sewage used for irrigation has been reported in literatures [5, 13, 47, 50, 53, 82, 92, 93]. In a study Mohamed et al. [12] reported that the copper content in vegetables of Saudi Arabia ranged between 0.43 mg kg^{-1} (in cabbages (*Brassica oleracea* var. *capitata* L.)) and 4.49 mg kg^{-1} (in green pepper (*Capsicum frutescens*)) (Table 2). Copper content in vegetables from Greece has been reported as 0.89-3.89 mg kg^{-1} in lettuce (*Lactuca sativa*), 0.17-0.41 mg kg^{-1} in carrots (*Daucas carota* L.), 0.26-1.03 mg kg^{-1} in cabbages (*Brassica oleracea* L.), 0.29-0.49 mg kg^{-1} in leek (*Allium ampeloprasum* var. *porrum* L.), and 0.44-0.72 mg kg^{-1} in endive (*Cichorium endivia*) (Table 3) [25]. A market basket survey showed that the copper content in vegetables from Pakistan ranged between 1.0±0.00 mg kg^{-1} (in radish (*Rapnus sativus* L.)) and 3.3±0.01 mg kg^{-1} (in mustard (*Brassica juncea*)) (Table 6) [76]. In Nigerian vegetables, copper content has been reported as 0.41 mg kg^{-1} in cabbage, 0.07 mg kg^{-1} in pumpkin leaves, 0.72 mg kg^{-1} in lettuce, 0.20 mg kg^{-1} in bitter leaf, 0.40 mg kg^{-1} in carrot, 0.36 mg kg^{-1} in tomatoes, 5.47 mg kg^{-1} in garden egg (*Solanum melongena*), 6.95 mg kg^{-1} in okra, and onion 7.30 mg kg^{-1} [94]. Onianwa et al. [94] reported that among different food groups in Nigeria the highest variation in Cu level was observed in leafy and fruity vegetables (about 169%), and the average level of Cu in this food group was 1.6±2.7 mg kg^{-1} (ranged between 0.07 and 7.30 mg kg^{-1}). However the Indian vegetables contain much higher amount of copper compared to other countries reported. Gupta et al. [66] reported that copper content in some common vegetables of India ranged between 13.4 mg kg^{-1} (in lettuce (*Lactuca sativa*)) and 48.6 mg kg^{-1} (in spinach (*Spinacia oleracea* L.)) (Table 5).

The recommended daily allowance for dietary copper is 2.5 mg day^{-1} [94-96]. Voutsa et al. [54] estimated the daily dietary intake of trace elements by the Greek population on the basis of the concentration of vegetable contaminants (dry weight), the percent moisture of vegetables (ranged between 90 and 95%), and of the daily availability of the specific vegetable species (the mean total daily availability of main foods, except water and beverages, per capita in Greece is 1575 g day^{-1} in which vegetables contribute about 15.3% (241 g day^{-1}) [97]). Voutsa et al. [54] determined trace elements in five common vegetables in Greece which account for 25.3% of the mean total vegetable consumption, that is 3.9% of the total food consumption. Accordingly the total dietary intake of Cu from those five vegetables was estimated to be 11-20 μg day^{-1} (mean daily availability of those five vegetables was 61 g), and if most of the vegetable in Greek diet have similar Cu content the total daily intake of Cu from vegetables was estimated to be 43-79 μg day^{-1} (mean daily availability of vegetables in Greek diet was 241 g (15.3% of the total diet) [97]).

Dietary intake of Cu in some countries of Asia, Europe, and North America has been reported in literature [94]. In Britain, Germany, and Hungary the daily dietary intake of Cu from all food sources were 1.51 mg (ranged between 1.25 and 3.1 mg), 2.7 mg (ranged between 0.6-12.3 mg), and 1.23 mg, respectively. In India and Japan the amount were 5.8 and 3.6 mg day^{-1}, respectively. In Russia, USA, and Canada the daily dietary intake of Cu were reported as 1.3-4.3, 0.76-1.7, and 2.2 mg, respectively [94]. But how much was the contribution of vegetables in total dietary intake of Cu for these countries is not clear. If we consider the contribution of vegetables in total daily diet for an adult in all countries as 15.3% (the daily availability of vegetables for a Greek adult in total diet is 241 g, which is 15.3% of total diet [54]), at least 0.23, 0.41, 0.88, 0.55, 0.19, and 0.34 mg of Cu day^{-1} would be consumed from vegetables by an adult in Britain, Germany, India, Japan, Russia, USA, and Canada, respectively.

The adult human body contains about 1.5±2.0 mg kg^{-1} of Cu which is essential as a constituent of some metalloenzymes and is required in haemoglobin synthesis and in the catalysis of metabolic oxidation [94]. The critical food Cu threshold for human health is 10 mg kg^{-1} [5]. Symptoms of copper deficiency in humans include bone demineralisation, depressed growth, depigmentation, and gastro-intestinal disturbances, among others, while toxicity due to excessive intake has been reported to cause liver cirrhosis, dermatitis and neurological disorders [98-100].

Lead (Pb)

Sources of human exposure:

Lead is commonly found in soil especially near roadways, older houses, old orchards, mining areas, industrial sites, near power plants, incinerators, landfills, and hazardous waste sites. People living near hazardous waste sites may be exposed to lead and chemicals that contain lead by breathing air, drinking water, eating foods, or swallowing dust or dirt that contain lead [101]. People living in areas where there are old houses that have been painted with lead paint may be exposed to higher levels of lead in dust and soil. Similarly, people who live near busy highways or on old orchard land where lead arsenate pesticides were used in the past may be exposed to higher levels of lead. People may also be exposed to lead when they work in jobs where lead is used or have hobbies in which lead is used, such as making stained glass [101].

One major source of environmental lead and of lead exposure to humans, both through direct inhalation and from ingestion following contamination of food chains, has been from the combustion of leaded petrol. Leafy fresh vegetables grown in lead-containing soils may have lead-containing dust on them. Lead may also enter foods if they are put into improperly glazed pottery or ceramic dishes and from leaded-crystal glassware [101].

Health effects:

In the human body, lead inhibits porphobilinogen synthase and ferrochelatase, preventing both porphobilinogen formation and the incorporation of iron into protoporphyrin IX, the final step in heme synthesis. This causes ineffective heme synthesis and subsequent microcytic anemia. At lower levels, it acts as a calcium analog, interfering with ion channels during nerve conduction. This is one of the mechanisms by which it interferes with cognition.

The main target for lead toxicity is the nervous system, both in adults and children. Long-term exposure of adults to lead at work has resulted in decreased performance in some tests that measure functions of the nervous system. Lead exposure may also cause weakness in fingers, wrists, or ankles. Lead exposure also causes small increases in blood pressure, particularly in middle-aged and older people. Lead exposure may also cause anemia. At high levels of exposure, lead can severely damage the brain and kidneys in adults or children and ultimately cause death. In pregnant women, high levels of exposure to lead may cause miscarriage. High level exposure in men can damage the organs responsible for sperm production [101].

Dietary intake:

Lead is generally considered to be only sparingly taken up and translocated to the edible tissues of vegetable crops [102]. Chumbley and Unwin [103] measured the Pb content in some common vegetable in Britain and reported that lettuce, cabbage, leek, onion, spinach, cauliflower, potato, radish, and sweet corn content 2.3-10.1, 0.3-0.8, 0.8-6.0, 0.6-1.5, 3.7-7.0, 2.0-7.1, 0.2-0.3, 2.9-4.9, and 0.1-0.2 mg kg^{-1} dry weight of Pb, respectively. Lead content in vegetables from Saudi Arabia has also been reported (Table 2) which show that the highest was 14.37 mg kg^{-1} in watercress (*Nasturtium officinale*, *N. microphyllum*) and the lowest was 2.59 mg kg^{-1} in tomato (*Lycopersicon esculentum* L.) [12]. In Greek vegetables, the Pb content ranged between 0.08-24.20 mg kg^{-1} dry weight (Table 3). It was reported that the lead contents in some common Greek vegetables; leek, carrot, lettuce, endive, and cabbage were 0.31-16.50, 0.08-0.71, 0.17-15.30, 1.42-24.20, and 0.49-15.50 mg kg^{-1} dry weight, respectively [25]. Bahemuka and Mubofu [13] reported lead content in some common leafy vegetables in Tanzania (Table 4) among which the highest was in cowpea leaves (6.6 mg kg^{-1} dry weight) and the lowest was in cabbage (1.90 mg kg^{-1} dry weight). Indian vegetables content much higher amount of lead compared to other countries. The lead content was highest in radish (50.0-63.5 mg kg^{-1} dry weight) while the lowest was in pudina (*Mentha arvensis*) (15.3-26.5 mg kg^{-1} dry weight) [66]. This amount was several times higher than the safe limit of Pb for human consumption (2.5 mg kg^{-1}).

Table 4: Heavy metal concentrations in some common vegetables of Tanzania [13].

Vegetables (Scientific Name)	Heavy metal content (mg kg^{-1})			
	Cd	Cu	Pb	Zn
Leafy cabbages (*Brassica oleracea* L.)	0.1	5.0-5.6	1.90-3.10	37.6-41.8
Cowpea leaves (*Vigna sinensis* L.)	0.2-0.6	8.5-9.1	2.8-6.6	33.6-34.6
Lettuce (*Lactuca sativa)*	0.3-0.4	2.5-5.8	3.6-3.8	14.8-15.9
African spinach (*Spinacia oleracea* L.)	0.3-0.6	7.2-13.7	3.0-5.9	40.8-48.1
Chinese cabbages (*Brassica chinensis* L.)	0.2	4.9-7.5	3.2-6.1	23.8-49.3
Pumpkin leaves (*Cucurbita moschata* L.)	0.2	9.4-16.0	3.4-3.9	27.7-36.7

Sapunar-Postruznik et al. [104] reported that the lead content in vegetables in the Republic of Croatia was 94 μg kg^{-1}. The general population of Croatia consumes an average of 274 g of vegetable day^{-1} and the intake of lead from vegetables was calculated to be about 25.85 μg $person^{-1}$ day^{-1}. Lead intake by a Greek adult has been reported as 0.8-26 μg day^{-1} from cabbage, 0.1-0.5 μg day^{-1} from carrot, 0.1-6.6 μg day^{-1} from leek, 0.2-14 μg day^{-1} from lettuce, and 3.4-58 μg day^{-1} from endive. Notably, the mean daily availability of cabbage, carrot, leek, lettuce, and endive for a Greek adult was estimated to be 17, 7, 4, 9, and 24, respectively [54]. It was estimated that the average daily dietary intake of lead from these five vegetables was 4.6-105 μg day^{-1}, and if all other Greek vegetables contain the similar amount of lead the total daily intake of the metal would be 18-415 μg day^{-1} (the mean daily vegetable availability for a Greek adult was 241 g [97]). However, the total intake of Pb from vegetables represents about 23.6% of the provisional tolerable daily intake [55]. Dietary intake of lead among the general population in Korea was reported to be 20.5 μg day^{-1} [105].

Zinc (Zn)

Sources of human exposure:

Zinc is one of the most common elements in the Earth's crust. Zinc is found in the air, soil, and water and is present in all foods. Zinc enters the air, water, and soil as a result of both natural processes and human activities. Most zinc enters the environment as the result of mining, purifying of zinc, lead, and cadmium ores, steel production, coal burning, and burning of wastes. These activities can increase zinc levels in the atmosphere. Waste streams from zinc and other metal manufacturing and zinc chemical industries, domestic waste water, and run-off from soil containing zinc can discharge zinc into waterways. The level of zinc in soil increases mainly from disposal of zinc wastes from metal manufacturing industries and coal ash from electric utilities. Sludge and fertilizer also contribute to increased levels of zinc in the soil [106].

Exposure of the general population to zinc is primarily by ingestion. The average daily intake of zinc from food in humans is 5.2–16.2 mg zinc/day; assuming a 70-kg average body weight, this corresponds to 0.07–0.23 mg zinc/kg/day [106]. Zinc is widespread in commonly consumed foods, but tends to be higher in those of animal origin, particularly some sea foods. Meat products contain relatively high concentrations of zinc, whereas fruits and vegetables have relatively low concentrations. Other possible pathways for zinc exposure are water and air. Individuals involved in galvanizing, smelting, welding, or brass foundry operations are exposed to metallic zinc and zinc compounds [106].

Health effects:

Zinc is an essential trace element, necessary for sustaining all plants and animals and is thought to protect plants from drought and disease. Zinc constitutes about 33 mg kg^{-1} of adult body weight and is essential as a constituent of many enzymes involved in a number of physiological functions, such as protein synthesis and energy metabolism [94]. Zn plays a fundamental role in expression of the genetic potential; the synthesis, repair and structural integrity of nucleic acids require Zn. Therefore, it is not surprising that deficiency of Zn reduces growth in almost all biological systems via decreased cell replication [107]. Zinc deficiency, resulting from poor diet, alcoholism and malabsorption, causes dwarfism, hypogonadism and dermatitis, while toxicity of zinc, due to excessive intake, may lead to electrolyte imbalance, nausea, anaemia and lethargy [107, 108]. Even though zinc is a very essential requirement for a healthy body, excess zinc can be harmful. Excessive absorption of zinc can also suppress copper and iron absorption. The free zinc ion in solution is highly toxic to plants, invertebrates, and even vertebrate fish. The Free Ion Activity Model (FIAM) is well-established in the literature, and shows that just micromole amount of the free ion kills some organisms. A recent example showed 6 micromole killing 93% of all *Daphnia* in water [109].

Dietary intake:

Although a variety of human diets contribute to the intake of Zn, however, vegetables are reported to be one of the important sources. Zinc contents in common vegetables of many countries have been reported by researchers. Mohamed et al. [12] investigated Zn content in some common vegetables in Saudi Arabia which show that watercress (*Nasturtium officinale, N. microphyllum*) had the highest amount of Zn (105.20 mg kg^{-1} dry weight) while the potato (*Solanum tuberosum* L.) had the lowest (4.50 mg kg^{-1} dry weight) (Table 2). Among the Greek vegetables about 20.10-140.00 mg kg^{-1} dry weight of Zn was found in endive (*Cichorium endivia*) while it was 8.90-40.50 in leek (*Allium ampeloprasum* var. *porrum* L.) (Table 3) [25]. In Tanzania, Zn contents were reported as 37.6-41.8 mg kg^{-1} in leafy cabbage (*Brassica oleracea var. capitata* L.), 14.8-15.9 mg kg^{-1} in lettuce (*Lactuca sativa*), 40.8-48.1 mg kg^{-1} in African spinach (*Spinacia oleracea* L.), 23.8-49.3 mg kg^{-1} in Chinese cabbage (*Brassica chinensis* L.), and 27.7-36.7 mg kg^{-1} in pumpkin leaves (*Cucurbita moschata* L.) (Table 4) [13]. Among south Asian countries Zn content in Pakistani vegetables have lower than that in Indian vegetables. The Zn content in Pakistani vegetables ranged between 0.1±0.00 and 1.2±0.01 mg kg^{-1} dry weight (Table 6) [76] while its content in Indian vegetables ranged between 82.6 and 193.7 mg kg^{-1} dry weight (Table 5)

[66]. Among the Indian vegetables the highest content of Zn (136.5-181.0 mg kg^{-1} dry weight) was observed in spinach (*Spinacia oleracea* L.) and the lowest (82.6-123.0 mg kg^{-1} dry weight) in cauliflower (*Brassica oleracea var. botrytis* L.). However, these values are much higher than the safe limit for human consumption (50.0 mg kg^{-1}) [66].

Table 5: Heavy metal concentrations in some common vegetables of India grown in waste-water irrigated agricultural soil [66].

Vegetables (Scientific Name)	Heavy metal Content (mg kg^{-1})				
	Cd	Cu	Cr	Pb	Zn
Pudina (*Mentha arvensis)*	5.4-31.0	18.7-30.7	58.4-75.3	15.3-26.5	110.9-153.0
Cauliflower(*Brassica oleracea* L.)	7.0-30.0	13.4-18.1	74.8-103.0	28.3-35.6	82.6-123.0
Lettuce (*Lactuca sativa)*	10.3-28.0	17.6-37.8	50.4-70.5	33.1-38.0	149.4-193.7
Spinach (*Spinacia oleracea* L.)	6.5-32.0	22.1-48.6	74.0-115.4	41.9-60.5	136.5-181.0
Chinese onion (*Allium cepa* L.)	5.7-25.0	16.3-18.9	40.3-53.2	22.8-41.4	110.9-150.0
Radish (*Rapnus sativus* L.)	11.8-28.6	18.7-35.1	69.8-100.0	50.0-63.5	125.4-157.3

Table 6: Concentration of heavy metals in vegetables procured from local markets of Pakistan [76].

Vegetable (Scientific Name)	Heavy metal Content (mg kg^{-1})		
	Cu	Zn	Cr
Lady finger (*Abelmoschus esculantus* L.)	1.8 ± 0.01	8.6 ± 0.04	0.7 ± 0.01
Pumpkin (*Cucurbita moschata* L.)	1.7 ± 0.01	4.1 ± 0.02	0.8 ± 0.02
Tomato (*Lycopersicon esculentum* L.)	1.3 ± 0.01	4.4 ± 0.03	0.5 ± 0.04
Brinjil (*Solanum melongena)*	3.1 ± 0.02	7.1 ± 0.05	0.7 ± 0.02
Potato (*Solanum tuberosum* L.)	1.2 ± 0.00	2.6 ± 0.01	0.3 ± 0.00
Beet (*Beta vulgaris)*	1.9 ± 0.01	3.6 ± 0.02	0.7 ± 0.02
Radish (*Rapnus sativus* L.)	1.0 ± 0.00	3.4 ± 0.02	0.5 ± 0.01
Carrot (*Daucas carota* L.)	1.2 ± 0.00	5.2 ± 0.04	0.8 ± 0.01
Turnip (*Brassica rapa* var. *rapa)*	1.1 ± 0.01	4.1 ± 0.02	0.4 ± 0.00
Mustard (*Brassica juncea)*	3.3 ± 0.01	5.4 ± 0.03	0.1 ± 0.00
Cabbage (*Brassica oleracea* L.)	1.1 ± 0.00	3.8 ± 0.02	0.4 ± 0.00
Spinach (*Spinacia oleracea* L.)	2.9 ± 0.01	6.1 ± 0.03	0.7 ± 0.02
Coriander (*Coriandrum sativum)*	1.8 ± 0.00	3.7 ± 0.04	1.2 ± 0.01

Recommended dietary allowances for Zn have been set at a level of 15 mg for adult males and 12 mg for adult non-pregnant and non-lactating women, based on an average requirement of 2.5 mg day^{-1} for absorbed Zn and an absorption efficiency of 20%, to meet the needs of all healthy persons, including those who consume diets with low Zn bioavailability [110]. High level of Zn in vegetables of many countries, especially in India, might contribute its intake in human through daily diet significantly. In Egyptian diet the average vegetable consumption is about 238±21.6 g (between 43.6 and 351 g) a day [110]. Hussein et al. [110] estimated that Zn content in Egyptian vegetables was 41.9 mg kg^{-1} and thus the daily dietary intake of Zn from vegetables would be 0.84-9.8 mg. This value is lower than the safe limit daily Zn intake (15 mg and 12 mg for adult male and female, respectively [110]).

Voutsa and Samara [54] investigated the Zn content in some common vegetables in Greece and estimated the daily dietary intake of the element in human. According to their estimation the mean daily dietary intake of Zn is 109 μg day^{-1} from cabbage, 15 μg day^{-1} from carrot, 9 μg day^{-1} from leek, 35 μg day^{-1} from lettuce, 59 μg day^{-1} from endive. Voutsa and Samara [54] also estimated that every day 61 g of these five vegetables are consumed by a Greek adult which contribute 227 μg of Zn. Moreover, the total daily vegetable consumption by Greek population is 241 g, and if all vegetables content similar amount of Zn the daily Zn intake would be 897 μg only from vegetables.

The vegetable consumption by Indian and other south Asian population is between 200 and 300 g day^{-1}. On the basis of Zn content in some common Indian vegetables reported in literature [66], the daily dietary intake of Zn by Indian population would be 16.52-58.11 mg. This amount is above the permissible limit of total Zn in daily diet (15 mg and 12 mg for adult male and female, respectively [110]).

Conclusion

Dietary intakes of toxic elements not only depend on the concentration of the elements in the vegetables but also evidently associated with the food habit and consumption rate by the population of a certain geographical area. Concentrations of some potentially toxic elements in a variety of vegetable species from different region of the world are compiled within the scope of the present article, and the dietary intake of the toxic elements in the vegetables for the corresponding region or country are discussed. Emphasis was given on data in available literatures and personal communication. Vegetables of south Asian countries like Bangladesh, India, and Pakistan have found to contain high level of toxic elements compared to other areas. Especially arsenic could be a major threat to the health of the population of this sub-continent. The food habit as well as the pattern of food consumption by the population of this area is also favorable in the dietary intake of toxic metals. Excessive use of contaminated groundwater in cooking and drinking could present a new dimension in health risk from arsenic in south Asia through the inclusion of arsenic in the food chains.

The contents of toxic elements in vegetables of some European countries were significantly lower then those in vegetables of south Asian and African countries. A detail discussion of the content of toxic elements in some common vegetables of Greece has been found in literatures which represents the European countries in this discussion. Data of Tanzania is considered as representative of African countries. Toxic elements in vegetables of Saudi Arabian markets have also been included in this discussion which might give an idea about the dietary intake of metals from vegetables of other Arabian countries. Considering the contents of toxic elements in vegetables of different areas worldwide, it can be concluded that vegetables could be a potential route for the dietary intake of those elements for the populations of highly contaminated areas.

References

[1] Sparks, DL. Toxic Metals in the Environment: The Role of Surfaces. *ELEMENTS*, 2005. 1, 193-197.

[2] Hillel, D. Heavy metals. In: Hillel, D, editor. *Encyclopedia of Soils in the Environment*. Amsterdam: Elsevier; 2005, 175-182.

[3] Roberts, DR; Nachtegaal, M; Sparks, DL. Speciation of metals in soils. In: Roberts, DR; Nachtegaal, M; Sparks, DL, editors. *Speciation of metals in soils*. Madison, WI.: Soil Science Society of America, 2005.

[4] Adriano, DC. Trace elements in the terestrial Environment. In: Adriano, DC, editor. *Trace elements in the terestrial Environment*. New york: Springer-Verlag, 2001.

[5] Islam, E; Yang, X-e; He, Z-l; Mahmood, Q. Assessing potential dietary toxicity of heavy metals in selected vegetables and food crops. *Journal of Zhejiang University (Science B)*, 2007. 8, 1-13.

[6] Sharma, RK; Agrawal, M; Marshall, FM. Heavy metal (Cu, Zn, Cd and Pb) contamination of vegetables in urban India: A case study in Varanasi *Environmental Pollution*, 2008. 154, 254-263.

[7] Åkesson, A; Julin, B; Wolk, A. Long-term Dietary Cadmium Intake and Postmenopausal Endometrial Cancer Incidence: A Population-Based Prospective Cohort Study. *Cancer Research*, 2008. 68, 6435-6441.

[8] Al Jassir, MS; Shaker, A; Khaliq, MA. Deposition of Heavy Metals on Green Leafy Vegerables Sold on Roadsides of Riyadh City, Saudi Arabia *Bulletin of Environmental Contamination and Toxicology*, 2005. 75, 1020-1027.

[9] Demirezen, D; Aksoy, A. Heavy Metal Levels in Vegetables in Turkey are within Safe Limits for Cu, Zn, Ni and exceeded for Cd and Pb. *Journal of Food Quality*, 2006. 29, 252-265.

[10] Gulz, PA; Gupta, S-K; Schulin, R. Arsenic accumulation of common plants from contaminated soils. *Plant and Soil*, 2005. 272, 337-347.

[11] Pillay, AE; Williams, JR; El Mardi, MO; Al-Lawati, SMH; Al-Hadabbi, MH; Al-Hamdi, A. Risk assessment of chromium and arsenic in date palm leaves used as livestock feed. *Environment International*, 2003. 29, 541-545.

[12] Mohamed, AE; Rashed, MN; Mofty, A. Assessment of essential and toxic elements in some kinds of vegetables. *Ecotoxicology and Environmental Safety*, 2003. 55, 251-260.

[13] Bahemuka, TE; Mubofu, EB. Heavy metals in edible green vegetables grown along the sites of the Sinza and Msimbazi rivers in Dar es Salaam, Tanzania. *Food Chemistry*, 1999. 66, 63-66.

[14] Hassan, N; Ahmad, K. Intra-familial distribution of food in rural Bangladesh. *Food and nutrition bulletin*, 1984. 6, 34-42.

[15] Khair, A. Vegetable. In: *Banglapedia: National Encyclopedia of Bangladesh [online edition]*. Islam, S, Editor. 2006, Asiatic Society of Bangladesh: Dhaka.

[16] Anonymous. In: Anonymous, editor. Dhaka, Bangladesh: Asiatic Society Bangladesh, 2006.

[17] Moriyama, N; Doyle, W. Women Don't Get Old or Fat: Secrets of My Mother's Tokyo Kitchen: Delacorte Press. 2005.

[18] Patterson, BH; Block, G. Food choices and the cancer guidelines. *Am J Public Health*, 1988. 78, 282-286.

[19] NRC. Diet and Health: Implications for Reducing Chronic Disease Risk. Washington, DC: National Academy Press. 1989.

[20] US Department of Agriculture, UDoHaHS. Nutrition and Your Health: Dietary Guidelines for Americans. Washington, DC: Govt Printing Office. 1980.

[21] Cronin, FJ; Shaw, AM; Krebs Smith, SM; Marsland, PM; Light, L. Developing a food guidance system to implement the dietary guidelines. *Journal of Nutritional Education*, 1987. 19, 281-302.

[22] Patterson, BH; Block, G; Rosenberger, WF; Pee, D; Kahle, LL. Fruit and vegetables in the American diet: data from the NHANES II survey. *Am J Public Health*, 1990. 80, 1443-1449.

[23] Knoops, KTB; de Groot, LCPGM; Kromhout, D; Perrin, A-E; Moreiras-Varela, O; Menotti, A; van Staveren, WA. Mediterranean Diet, Lifestyle Factors, and 10-Year Mortality in Elderly European Men and Women: The HALE Project. *JAMA*, 2004. 292, 1433-1439.

[24] Lake, DL; Kirk, PWW; Lester, JN. Fractionation, Characterization, and Speciation of Heavy Metals in Sewage Sludge and Sludge-Amended Soils: A Review. *J Environ Qual*, 1984. 13, 175-183.

[25] Voutsa, D; Grimanis, A; Samara, C. Trace elements in vegetables grown in an industrial area in relation to soil and air particulate matter. *Environmental Pollution*, 1996. 94, 325-335.

[26] Zurera-Cosano, G; Moreno-Rojas, R; Salmeron-Egea, J; Pozo Lora, R. Heavy metal uptake from greenhouse border soils for edible vegetables. *Journal of the Science of Food and Agriculture*, 1989. 49, 307-314.

[27] Pinochet, H; De Gregori, I; Lobos, MG; Fuentes, E. Selenium and Copper in Vegetables and Fruits Grown on Long-Term Impacted Soils from Valparaiso Region, Chile. *Bulletin of Environmental Contamination and Toxicology*, 1999. 63, 327-334.

[28] Stalikas, CD; Mantalovas, AC; Pilidis, GA. Multielement concentrations in vegetable species grown in two typical agricultural areas of Greece. *Science of The Total Environment*, 1997. 206, 17-24.

[29] Ursinyova, M; Hladikova, V; Uhnak, J; Kovacicova, J. Toxic elements in environmental samples from selected regions in Slovakia. *Bulletin of Environmental Contamination and Toxicology ; VOL. 58 ; ISSUE: 6 ; PBD: Jun 1997*, 1997, pp. 985-992 ; PL:.

[30] WHO. Evaluation of certain food additives and contaminants. In: *61st report of the Joint FAO/WHO Expert Committee on Food Additives*. World Health Organization (WHO): Geneva. 1993.

[31] Wolnik, KA; Fricke, FL; Capar, SG; Braude, GL; Meyer, MW; Satzger, RD; Kuennen, RW. Elements in major raw agricultural crops in the United States. 2. Other elements in lettuce, peanuts, potatoes, soybeans, sweet corn, and wheat. *Journal of Agricultural and Food Chemistry*, 1983. 31, 1244-1249.

[32] Wolnik, KA; Fricke, FL; Capar, SG; Meyer, MW; Satzger, RD; Bonnin, E; Gaston, CM. Elements in major raw agricultural crops in the United States. 3. Cadmium, lead,

and eleven other elements in carrots, field corn, onions, rice, spinach, and tomatoes. *Journal of Agricultural and Food Chemistry*, 1985. 33, 807-811.

[33] Rashed, MN; R M Awadallah. Trace elements in faba bean (<I>Vicia faba</I>L) plant and soil as determined by atomic absorption spectroscopy and ion selective electrode. *Journal of the Science of Food and Agriculture*, 1998. 77, 18-24.

[34] Samara, C; Misaelides, P; Tsalev, D; Anousis, I; Kouimtzis, T. Trace element distribution in vegetables grown in the industrial area of Thessaloniki/Greece. *Fresenius Environmental Bulletin*, 1992. . 1, 577-582.

[35] Gerberding, JL. Toxicological Profile for Arsenic. Agency for Toxic Substances and Disease Registry (ATSDR): Atlanta, Georgia 2007.

[36] Chen, CJ; Wu, MM; Lee, SS. Atherogenicity and carcinogenicity of high arsenic artesian well water: multiple risk factors and related malignant neoplasms of blackfoot disease. *Arteriosclerosis, Thrombosis, and Vascular Biology*, 1988. 8, 452-460.

[37] Guha Mazumder, DN; Haque, R; Ghosh, N; De, BK; Santra, A; Chakraborty, D; Smith, AH. Arsenic levels in drinking water and the prevalence of skin lesions in West Bengal, India. *International Journal of Epidemiology*, 1998. 27, 871-877.

[38] Maharjan, M; Watanabe, C; Ahmad, SA; Umezaki, M; Ohtsuka, R. Mutual interaction between nutritional status and chronic arsenic toxicity due to groundwater contamination in an area of Terai, lowland Nepal. *Journal of Epidemiology and Community Health*, 2007. 61, 389-394.

[39] Mitra, SR; Guha Mazumder, DN; Basu, A. Nutritional factors and susceptibility to arsenic-caused skin lesions in West Bengal, India. *Environmental Health Perspectives*, 2004. 112, 1104-1109.

[40] Smith, AH; Smith, MMH. Arsenic drinking water regulations in developing countries with extensive exposure. *Toxicology*, 2004. 198, 39-44.

[41] Smith, AH; Arroyo, AP; Guha Mazumder, DN. Arsenic-induced skin lesions among Atacameno people in Northern Chile despite good nutrition and centuries of exposure. *Environmental Health Perspectives*, 2000. 108, 617-620.

[42] Milton, AH; Hasan, Z; Shahidullah, SM. Association between nutritional status and arsenicosis due to chronic arsenic exposure in Bangladesh. *International Journal of Environmental Health Research*, 2004. 14, 99-108.

[43] Dabeka, RW; McKenzie, AD; Lacroix, GMA; Cleroux, C; Bowe, S; Graham, RA; Conacher, HBS; Verdier, P. Survey of arsenic in Total Diet food composites and estimation of the dietary intake of arsenic by Canadian adults and children. *Journal of AOAC INTERNATIONAL*, 1993. 76, 14-25.

[44] Schoof, RA; Yost, LJ; Eickhoff, J; Crecelius, EA; Cragin, DW; Meacher, DM; Menzel, DB. A Market Basket Survey of Inorganic Arsenic in Food. *Food and Chemical Toxicology*, 1999. 37, 839-846.

[45] Urieta, I; Jalon, M; Eguileor, I. Food surveillance in the Basque country (Spain). II. Estimation of the dietary intake of organochlorine pesticides, heavy metals, arsenic, aflatoxin M1, ironand zinc through the Total Diet Study, 1990/91. *Food Additives and Contaminants*, 1996. 13, 29-52.

[46] Ysart, G; Miller, P; Crews, H; Robb, P; Baxter, M; De L'Argy, C; Lofthouse, S; Sargent, C; Harrison, N. Dietary exposure estimates of 30 elements from the UK Total Diet Study. *Food Additives and Contaminants*, 1999. 16, 391-403.

[47] MAFF. Total Diet Study: aluminium, arsenic, cadmium, chromium, copper, lead, mercury, nickel, selenium, tin and zinc. Food surveillance information sheet, No. 191. Ministry of Agriculture, Fisheries and Food (MAFF): HMSO, London, U.K. 1997.

[48] Sapunar-Postruznik, J; Bazulic, D; Kubala, H. Estimation of dietary intake of arsenic in the general population of the Republic of Croatia. *The Science of The Total Environment*, 1996. 191, 119-123.

[49] Rahman, IMM; Nazim Uddin, M; Hasan, MT; Hossain, MM. Assimilation of arsenic into edible plants grown in soil irrigated with contaminated groundwater. In: Rahman, IMM; Nazim Uddin, M; Hasan, MT; Hossain, MM, editors. *Natural Arsenic in Groundwaters of Latin America*. London, UK: Taylor and Francis; 2008, 351-358.

[50] Buchet, JP; Lauwerys, R; Vanderwoorde, A; Pycke, JM. Oral daily intake of cadmium, lead, manganese, copper, chromium, chromium, mercury, calcium, zinc and arsenic in Belgium: a duplicate meal study. *Food and Chemical Toxicology*, 1983. 21, 19-24.

[51] De Vos, RH; Van Dokkum, W; Olthof, PDA; Quirijns, JK; Muys, T; Van der Poll, JM. Pesticides and other chemical residues in Dutch total diet samples (June 1976-July 1978). *Food and Chemical Toxicology*, 1984. 22, 11-21.

[52] Jorhem, L; Becker, W; Slorach, S. Intake of 17 Elements by Swedish Women, Determined by a 24-h Duplicate Portion Study. *Journal of Food Composition and Analysis*, 1998. 11, 32-46.

[53] Tsuda, T; Inoue, T; Kojima, M; Aoki, S. Market basket and duplicate portion estimation of dietary intakes of cadmium, mercury, arsenic, copper, manganese, and zinc by Japanese adults. *Journal of AOAC INTERNATIONAL*, 1995. 78, 1363-1368.

[54] Voutsa, D; Samara, C. Dietary intake of trace elements and polycyclic aromatic hydrocarbons via vegetables grown in an industrial Greek area. *The Science of The Total Environment*, 1998. 218, 203-216.

[55] WHO. Trace elements in human nutrition and health. Geneva: World Health Organization. 1996.

[56] USEPA. Special Report on Ingested Inorganic Arsenic. Skin Cancer, Nutritional Essentiality In: *(EPA/625/3-87/013)*. 1988, Environmental Protection Agency: Washington, DC.

[57] Chowdhury, UK; Rahman, MM; Mandal, BK; Paul, K; Lodh, D; Biswas, BK; Basu, GK; Chanda, CR; Saha, KC; Mukherjee, SC; Roy, S; Das, R; Kaies, I; Barua, AK; Palit, SK; Quamruzzaman, Q; Chakraborti, D. Groundwater arsenic contamination and human suffering in West Bengal, India and Bangladesh. *Environ. Sci.*, 2001. 8, 393-415.

[58] Tao, SH; Bolger, PM. Dietary intakes of arsenic in the United States. In: *3rd International Conference on Arsenic Exposure and Health Effects*. 1998: San Diego, CA.

[59] WHO. Inorganic arsenic compounds other than arsine: health and safety guide. In: *Health and safety guide; no. 70*. 1992, World Health Organization: Geneva.

[60] Cusack, P; Perrett, T. The EU RoHS Directive and its implications for the plastics industry. *Plastics, Additives and Compounding*, 2006. 8, 46-49.

[61] USEPA. *EPA Summary on Cadmium Compounds*. 2007 November 7 [cited 2009 January 20].

[62] Gerberding, JL. Toxicological Profile for Cadmium. Agency for Toxic Substances and Disease Registry (ATSDR): Atlanta, Georgia. 2008.

[63] Wallace, HA. Principles and Methods of Toxicology. In: Wallace, HA, editor. *Principles and Methods of Toxicology*. Philadelphia: Taylor and Francis Publishing Inc., 2001.

[64] Friberg, L. Cadmium. *Annual Review of Public Health*, 1983. 4, 367-367.

[65] Nogawa, K; Kobayashi, E; Okubo, Y; Suwazono, Y. Environmental cadmium exposure, adverse effects and preventive measures in Japan. *BioMetals*, 2004. 17, 581-587.

[66] Gupta, N; Khan, DK; Santra, SC. An Assessment of Heavy Metal Contamination in Vegetables Grown in Wastewater-Irrigated Areas of Titagarh, West Bengal, India *Bulletin of Environmental Contamination and Toxicology*, 2008. 80, 115-118.

[67] Reilly, C. Metal cotamination of foods: Its significance for food quality and human health In: Reilly, C, editor. *Metal cotamination of foods: Its significance for food quality and human health* London: Blackwell Science, 1991.

[68] Katz, SA; Salem, H. The biological and environmental chemistry of chromium. New York (USA): VCH Publishers. 1994.

[69] Koplan, JP. Toxicological profile for chromium. Agency for Toxic Substances and Disease Registry: Atlanta, Georgia. 2000.

[70] Becquer, T; Quantin, C; Sicot, M; Boudot, JP. Chromium availability in ultramafic soils from New Caledonia. *The Science of The Total Environment*, 2003. 301, 251-261.

[71] Huffman, EWD; Allaway, WH. Chromium in plants. Distribution in tissues, organelles, and extracts and availability of bean leaf chromium to animals. *Journal of Agricultural and Food Chemistry*, 1973b. 21, 982-986.

[72] Huffman, EWD, Jr.; Allaway, WH. Growth of Plants in Solution Culture Containing Low Levels of Chromium. *Plant Physiol.*, 1973a. 52, 72-75.

[73] Davies, FT; Puryear, JD; Newton, RJ; Egilla, JN; Grossi, JAS. Mycorrhizal Fungi Increase Chromium Uptake by Sunflower Plants: Influence on Tissue Mineral Concentration, Growth, and Gas Exchange. *Journal of Plant Nutrition*, 2002. 25, 2389 - 2407.

[74] Davies, JFT; Puryear, JD; Newton, RJ; Egilla, JN; Saraiva Grossi, JA. Mycorrhizal fungi enhance accumulation and tolerance of chromium in sunflower (Helianthus annuus). *Journal of Plant Physiology*, 2001. 158, 777-786.

[75] Shanker, AK; Cervantes, C; Loza-Tavera, H; Avudainayagam, S. Chromium toxicity in plants. *Environment International*, 2005. 31, 739-753.

[76] Hashmi, DR; Ismail, S; Shaikh, GH. Assessment of the level of trace metals in commonly edible vegetables locally available in the markets of Karachi city. *Pakistan Journal of Botany*, 2007. 39, 747-751.

[77] Ducros, V. Chromium metabolism. *Biological Trace Element Research*, 1992. 32, 65-77.

[78] Biego, GH; Joyeux, M; Hartemann, P; Debry, G. Daily intake of essential minerals and metallic micropollutants from foods in France. *The Science of The Total Environment*, 1998. 217, 27-36.

[79] NAS. Recommended dietary allowances. National Academy of Sciences: Washington DC. 1980.

[80] Anderson, R; Bryden, N; Polansky, M. Dietary chromium intake. *Biological Trace Element Research*, 1992. 32, 117-121.

[81] Van Cauwenbergh, R; Hendrix, P; Robberecht, H; Deelstra, HA. Daily dietary chromium intake in Belgium, using duplicate portion sampling. *Zeitschrift für Lebensmitteluntersuchung und -Forschung A*, 1996. 203, 203-206.

[82] Gaw, SK; N.D. Kim; G.L. Northcott; A.L. Wilkins; Robinson, G. Uptake of EDDT, Arsenic, Cadmium, Copper, and Lead by Lettuce and Radish Grown in Contaminated Horticultural Soils. *Journal of Agricultural and Food Chemistry*, 2008. 56, 6584-6593.

[83] Wong, MH; Bradshaw, AD. A Comparison of the Toxicity of Heavy Metals, Using Root Elongation of Rye Grass, Lolium Perenne. *New Phytologist*, 1982. 91, 255-261.

[84] Tianyu Li, ZX. A novel response of wild-type duckweed (*Lemna paucicostata* Hegelm.) to heavy metals. *Environmental Toxicology*, 2004. 19, 95-102.

[85] Gerberding, JL. Toxicological profile for copper. Agency for Toxic Substances and Disease Registry (ATSDR): Atlanta, Georgia. 2004.

[86] Araya, M; Chen, B; Klevay, LM; Strain, JJ; Johnson, L; Robson, P; Shi, W; Nielsen, F; Zhu, H; Olivares, M; Pizarro, F; Haber, LT. Confirmation of an acute no-observed-adverse-effect and low-observed-adverse-effect level for copper in bottled drinking water in a multi-site international study. *Regulatory Toxicology and Pharmacology*, 2003a. 38, 389-399.

[87] Araya, M; McGoldrick, MC; Klevay, LM; Strain, JJ; Robson, P; Nielsen, F; Olivares, M; Pizarro, F; Johnson, L; Poirier, KA. Determination of an Acute No-Observed-Adverse-Effect Level (NOAEL) for Copper in Water. *Regulatory Toxicology and Pharmacology*, 2001. 34, 137-145.

[88] Araya, M; Olivares, M; Pizarro, F; Gonzalez, M; Speisky, H; Uauy, R. Gastrointestinal symptoms and blood indicators of copper load in apparently healthy adults undergoing controlled copper exposure. *American Journal of Clinical Nutrition*, 2003b. 77, 646-650.

[89] Araya, M; Olivares, M; Pizarro, F; Mendez, MA; Gonzalez, M; Uauy, R. Supplementing copper at the upper level of the adult dietary recommended intake induces detectable but transient changes in healthy adults. *Journal of Nutrition*, 2005. 135, 2367-2371.

[90] Araya, M; Peña, C; Pizarro, F; Olivares, M. Gastric response to acute copper exposure. *The Science of The Total Environment*, 2003c. 303, 253-257.

[91] Araya, M; Manuel, O; Fernando, P. Copper in human health. *International Journal of Environment and Health*, 2007. 1, 608 - 620

[92] Beavington, F. Heavy metal contamination of vegetables and soil in domestic gardens around a smelting complex. *Environmental Pollution*, 1975. 9, 211-217.

[93] He, ZL; Yang, XE; Stoffella, PJ. Trace elements in agroecosystems and impacts on the environment. *Journal of Trace Elements in Medicine and Biology*, 2005. 19, 125-140

[94] Onianwa, PC; Adeyemo, AO; Idowu, OE; Ogabiela, EE. Copper and zinc contents of Nigerian foods and estimates of the adult dietary intakes. *Food Chemistry*, 2001. 72, 89-95.

[95] WHO. Trace element in human nutrition. In: *WHO Technical Report Series No.532*. World Health Organization: Geneva. 1973.

[96] WHO. Guidelines for the study of dietary intakes of chemical contaminants. In: *WHO Offset Publication No. 87*. World Health Organization: Geneva. 1985.

[97] Trichopoulou, A; Vassilakou, T. Food availability in greece per capita. Athens: Greek Society of Nutrition and Foods. 1995.

[98] Graham, GG; Cordano, A. Copper defciency in human subjects In: Graham, GG; Cordano, A, editors. *Copper defciency in human subjects* New York: Academic Press, 1976.

[99] Lucas, J. Our polluted food, a survey of the risks. New York: John Wiley and Sons. 1974.

[100] Somers, E. The toxic potential of trace metals in foods. A review. *Journal of Food Science*, 1974. 39, 215-217.

[101] Gerberding, JL. Toxicological Profile for Lead. Agency for Toxic Substances and Disease Registry (ATSDR): Atlanta, Georgia. 2007.

[102] DOE. Lead in the environment and its significance to man. Environment, Dot, Editor. 1974, HMSO: London.

[103] Chumbley, CG; Unwin, RJ. Cadmium and lead content of vegetable crops grown on land with a history of sewage sludge application *Environmental Pollution Series B, Chemical and Physical*, 1982. 4, 231-237.

[104] Sapunar-Postruznik, J; Bazulic, D; Kubala, H; Balint, L. Estimation of dietary intake of lead and cadmium in the general population of the Republic of Croatia. *Science of The Total Environment*, 1996. 177, 31-35.

[105] Moon, CS; Zhang, ZW; Shimbo, S; Watanabe, T; Moon, DH; Lee, CU; Lee, BK; Ahn, KD; Lee, SH; Ikeda, M. Dietary Intake of Cadmium and Lead among the General Population in Korea. *Environmental Research*, 1995. 71, 46-54.

[106] Gerberding, JL. Toxicological Profile for Zinc. Agency for Toxic Substances and Disease Registry (ATSDR): Atlanta, Georgia. 2005, p. 1-301.

[107] Fairweather-Tait, SJ. Zinc in Human Nutrition. *Nutrition Research Reviews*, 1988. 1, 23-37.

[108] Prasad, SA. Discovery and importance of zinc in human nutrition. *Federation Proceedings*, 1984. 43, 2829-2834.

[109] Muyssen, BTA; De Schamphelaere, KAC; Janssen, CR. Mechanisms of chronic waterborne Zn toxicity in Daphnia magna. *Aquatic Toxicology*, 2006. 77, 393-401.

[110] Hussein, L; Bruggeman, J. Zinc analysis of Egyptian foods and estimated daily intakes among an urban population group. *Food Chemistry*, 1997. 58, 391-398.

In: Fruit and Vegetable Consumption and Health
Editors: Anton Papareschi and Harvey Eppolito
ISBN: 978-1-60741-596-1

Chapter III

Determinants of Vegetable and Fruit Consumption among Mexican Children and Their Parents

Ana Bertha Pérez-Lizaur [a]***, Martha Kaufer-Horwitz*** [b*]***,***
Maite Plazas [c]***, Magdalena Vázquez*** [d]
and Mónica Pérez Lizaur [e]
[a] Universidad Iberoamericana, Mexico City, Mexico
[b] Instituto Nacional de Ciencias Médicas y Nutrición Salvador Zubirán, Mexico
[c] Ogali Consultoría en Nutrición, Mexico
[d] Independent Consultant, Mexico
[e] Independent Consultant, Mexico

Abstract

Background: Epidemiological evidence suggests that populations with high vegetable and fruit (VF) consumption (>5 portions/day) have a lower risk of developing childhood obesity, cancer, and cardiovascular diseases. In Mexico there is a dearth of information that identifies the determinants of VF intake in children. The aim of the present study was to assess the number of portions consumed by and the determinants of VF intake among children and their parents in a sample of Mexico City's public schools.

Methods: We administered two previously tested and validated questionnaires for children and their parents (Cronbach's *alpha* 0.84 and 0.74) respectively. We also administered a validated two-day dietary recall used to assess VF intake and its correlates among 327 children and a group of 142 parents.

* Correspondence: Please address correspondence to: Martha Kaufer-Horwitz DSc, Clínica de Obesidad y Trastornos de Alimentación. Instituto Nacional de Ciencias Médicas y Nutrición Salvador Zubirán. Vasco de Quiroga No. 15. Col. Sección XVI. Mexico D.F., 14000. Mexico. Phone: +52/55/ 54 87 09 00 Ext. 5068. Fax: +52/55/ 5513 9272. E-mail: marthakaufer@aol.com

Results: Among study participant, children consumed approximately one portion of VF per day. Girls consumed more VF than boys ($p<0.01$). Parents consumed four daily portions. Environmental factors that influenced a higher consumption of VF among children include: mothers being in charge of cooking the meals at home ($p<0.02$) and accessibility to VF (<0.01). Personal variables were self-efficacy ($p<0.05$) and vegetable preference ($p<0.03$). Being a girl (OR 2.2, CI: 1.04-4.7), accessibility to VF (OR 3.38, CI: 1.26-9.0) and total VF consumption among parents (OR 1.37, CI:1.08-1.7) were the determinants of VF consumption in the multivariate analysis. The personal and environmental factors that influenced a higher VF consumption among parents were knowledge ($p<0.05$) and vegetable preference (<0.01). Knowledge (OR 1.63, CI: 1.23-2.17) was the determinant of VF consumption among parents in the multivariate model.

Conclusion: The characteristics that correlate with VF consumption among children attending Mexico City's public school system include, being a girl, accessibility to VF and total VF consumption in parents. VF consumption for parents was correlated with knowledge. These factors should be considered when designing public policies aimed increasing VF consumption among children and their parents.

Keywords: fruit and vegetables, correlates, determinants, children, parents, Mexican, accessibility

Introduction

Epidemiological and experimental evidence suggest that populations with a high consumption of vegetables and fruit (VF) (>5 servings per day) have a lower risk for developing obesity (Rolls et al., 2004; Carlton et al., 2004; Sichieri, 2002), cancer (Riboli and Norat, 2003; Voorips et al., 2000; Hayes, 2005) and cardiovascular diseases (Bazzano et al., 2002; Colgan et al., 2004; Liu et al., 2000).

Various international health organizations (Aranceta and Serra Majem, 2001) recommend that in a healthy diet at least five servings of VF (400 to 500 g) be consumed per day (AICR, 1997; World Health Organization, 2003; Euro Diet, 2001); for children, serving sizes will be appropriately smaller. In Mexico, the Official Mexican Norm on Nutrition Education to the Public recommends the consumption of VF (Norma Oficial Mexicana, 2004), although the official guidelines do not include a specific recommendation on the number of daily portions.

Factors That Influence Food Consumption

The factors that influence food selection are not restricted to personal preferences; they are also conditioned by social, cultural, and financial circumstances (EUFIC, 2004), food cost, accessibility, and the lack of knowledge to design a healthy diet (Dibsdall et al., 2003; Satia et al., 2002). According to some authors, social groups with low purchasing power have a greater tendency to consume an unhealthy diet and fewer VF (<5 servings/day) (De Irala-Estevez et al., 2000) while others suggest that healthy diets are more expensive than those high in sugars, fat, and refined cereals (Drewnowski and Barratt-Fornell, 2003).

Eating habits that are acquired during childhood may persist into adulthood (Branen and Fletcher, 1999); therefore, factors that influence food consumption should be identified in order to carry out more effective interventions that will promote a healthy diet during the entire lifespan (Baranowski et al., 1997; Pérez et al., 2004).

With regards to the influence of familial variables, Cooke (2007) found that parents' food preferences are highly associated with their consumption patterns. Identifying the factors that influence food preferences are crucial to design effective public health interventions to improve children's diet. It is possible that one of the most important determinants of a child`s preference towards a certain food is its degree of familiarity with it. According to this author, "*In simple terms, children like what they know and eat what they like*".

It is well known that parents play a very important role in the development of their children's food preferences as well as in their caloric intake (Scaglioni, 2008). According to a study by Elfhag (2008) parents' food consumption is the most important characteristic that determines childrens' consumption when compared with any other variable. Sylvestre MP et al.,(2007) has suggested that in order to improve FV consumption we need to raise consciousness among parents about the importance of consuming FV and the impact their own behavior has on their children's consumption patterns.

A number of behavioral theories are applied to eating habits' research to describe the mechanisms by which attitudes and beliefs exert their influence on eating behavior (Glanz et al., 1997; Satia et al., 2002). It is expected that the efficiency and efficacy of individual and community interventions of health programs, particularly food programs, would increase as our understanding of basic behavioral mechanisms through these theories also increases. The Social Cognitive Theory (Bandura, 2001) proposes that an individual's behavior and environmental and personal characteristics interact in reciprocal relations (reciprocal determination), explaining the subject's behavior. This characteristics are defined as: accessibility (easiness with which the students were able to find ready-to-eat VF); expectancy (value that the person places on a given outcome); self-efficacy (the person's confidence in performing a particular behavior and in overcoming barriers to that behavior); preference (what the child likes to eat) and knowledge (what the child knows about the function of VF in the body) (Baranowski, 2002). Cullen´s group (Cullen et al., 2000) proposes applying this theory to nutrition education, as it has been successfully used as the foundation in health education interventions in schools (Klepp et al., 2005).

The intake of VF among Mexican children attending the public health system is not known. On the other hand, VF intake[1] among the adult population is considered insufficient for having a healthy diet and preventing chronic diseases. According to published international studies, nutrition education programs for children must include a number of key elements in order to achieve successful outcomes. These programs must be based on behavior and environmental modifications, involve the family when the children are young, engage the school to modify its environment, embrace the community, and include sufficient time to instruct program participants. In order to achieve a successful outcome, we need to

[1] One portion is includes ½ cup of vegetable or fruit juice or a medium size unit of fruit or vegetable (excluding potatoes).

understand the way in which these factors interact with the target population. The psychosocial characteristics of Mexican children associated with VF consumption have not been identified, and these are needed to carry out communication and food orientation campaigns that would promote greater intake of these food types in our country. Therefore, the aim of our study was to identify the number of servings of VF schoolchildren eat and the determinants of VF intake among Mexican children attending an urban school setting. We were also interested in describing the determinants of VF consumption among parents. With this information at hand, we would be able to assess the parent's and children's determinants of VF consumption which could serve as the basis for intervention programs.

Methods

The study was observational and cross-sectional. A total of 327 children (49.2% males and 50.8% females) attending second, third and fourth grade of primary school, with a mean age of 8.8 years (6-10 yrs) were recruited from one of Mexico City's public school districts (Alvaro Obregón). A sample of 142 parents were selected and agreed to participate in the study. The mean age for fathers was 36.0 years (SD ± 6.4) and 33.1 years (SD ± 5.46) for mothers. The parents' mean level of schooling was 8±3.5 years.

Families belonged to a low socioeconomic strata (AMAI 2004[2]), knew how to read and write. Once the study methodology was explained by members of the research team, they agreed to participate in the study and signed the informed consent form. Consent for study participation was obtained from the parents or guardians as well as from the school authorities. The study was approved by the corresponding Ethics Committee.

Two ad-hoc self-administered written questionnaires (one for children and one for parents) to identify environmental (accessibility and person in charge of cooking at home) and personal characteristics (preferences, expectancy, knowledge, and self-efficacy) that influence VF consumption among study participants were designed based on the experience of other investigators (Baranowski et al., 1997) and adapted to the study population. The children's questionnaire was administered during school hours and supervised by the study team. Parents completed the questionnaire at home. A pilot study was conducted to assess the instrument's internal validity. The score for the Cronbach *alpha* coefficient (Streiner and Norman, 2000; Prieto and Badia, 2001) for the children's questionnaire was 0.84, so its internal validity was accepted *a priori.* The *alpha* score for the parents' questionnaire was 0.74, also considered a reliable measuring instrument. The instrument included a validated two-day (Gunde, 2002) dietary recall (The children and their parents completed the dietary assessment component twice, once Wednesday to recall Tuesday and again on Saturday to recall Friday consumption. Each mention of a vegetable or a fruit in the written recall was defined as one serving, regardless of its size; for example, if the child mentioned spinach, it was considered one serving. Commercial fruit juices were not considered as fruits, because

[2] Families where the parents had completed primary and/or secondary school, live in a house with two rooms, and report a monthly income of approximately $250 US dollars per month.

of the sugar added to many commercial juices. Questions about number of hours of TV viewing and video games were also asked. Children's height and weight were measured in duplicate by trained personnel (Lohman et al., 1988). Overweight and obesity was defined as a Body Mass Index (BMI) greater than the 85th percentile of BMI for age and gender according to the National Center for Health Statistics tables (NCHS, 2000; Must, 1991). The results of this study have been published elsewhere and are partially described in this paper. (Pérez-Lizaur et al., 2008).

Statistical Methods

The children's (sample 1) and the parents' (sample 2) samples were analyzed separately. In the children's sample (sample 1) VF intake was considered as the dependent variable. The independent variables included: gender, personal characteristics (high self-efficacy, high expectancy, high preferences, and high knowledge) and environmental characteristics (high accessibility and person in charge of cooking at home). Personal characteristics and accessibility were divided into high and low, according to the group's median for each variable. In the parents' sample (sample 2) VF consumption among parents and their children was analyzed and two different analyses were carried out. In the first case, VF consumption among parents was considered the dependent variable and in the second case, VF consumption among children. In both cases, independent variables included personal and environmental variables reported by the parents. Also, when analyzing VF consumption among children, parents' consumption was also included. Children's VF consumption was divided into two groups: 2 or fewer servings per day and 3 or more servings per day (subsequently referred to as higher consumption). VF consumption among parents was also divided into two groups: 3 or fewer servings per day and 4 or more servings per day (subsequently referred to as higher consumption). Chi square (χ^2) tests were used to evaluate the association of the independent variables with VF intake. Variables with predictive value for VF intake were identified. Stepwise logistic regression was used to identify the correlates of higher VF consumption. Odds ratios were calculated with a 95% confidence interval. SPSS v12.0 was used for the analysis.

Results

Sample 1

The median intake of VF among children was 1 (0 to 5) servings per day, with only 25% of the children eating 3 or more servings of VF per day. When compared by gender, a significant difference was found in the VF consumption of girls and boys ($p< 0.01$). A higher proportion of girls consumed 3 or more servings per day (15.2%) compared with boys (6.7%) (Table 1).

Approximately 25% of study participants indicated that they had never tasted the VF listed in the questionnaire; 33% said they did not like them; and the remainder said they liked them. In relation to the BMI for age, 63.6% of the boys and 51.5% of the girls in the study were at risk for overweight or obesity, (χ^2 = 4.826; p< 0.03). About 41% of the children watched four or more hours of TV or video games a day.

Table 1. Gender distribution of study participants based on servings of vegetables and fruit consumption

Gender	Vegetable and fruit consumption		Total n (%)
	Two or less n (%)	Three or more n (%)	
Boy	152 (93.3%)	11 (6.7%)	163 (100 %)
Girl	139 (84.8%)	25 (15.2%)	164 (100 %)
Total	291 (89.0%)	36 (11.0%)	327 (100 %)

χ^2 = 6.022; p< 0.01

Table 2. Children's personal and environmental characteristics[3] that correlate with vegetable and fruit consumption

Determinants	Vegetable and fruit intake		Total n / N (327) n (%)	Statistical significance
	Lower 2 or less servings N=291 (%)	Higher 3 or more servings N=36 (%)		
Personal				
Gender				
Boy	152 (52.2)	11 (30.6)	163 (49.8%)	p= 0.07
Girl	139 (47.8)	25 (69.4)	164 (50.2%)	p<0.01
High knowledge	218 (74.9)	24 (66.7)	242 (74.0%)	p= 0.19
High preference for fruit	134 (46.0)	9 (25.0)	143 (43.7%)	p= 0.39
High preference for vegetables	130 (44.7%)	18 (50%)	148 (45.3%)	p= 0.34
High expectancy	159 (54.6)	23 (63.4)	182 (55.6%)	p= 0.19
High self-efficacy for vegetables	177 (60.8)	28 (77.8)	205 (62.7%)	p<0.05
High self-efficacy for fruits	196 (67.4)	27 (75.0)	223 (68.2%)	p= 0.23
ENVIRONMENTAL				
Mother cooks	239 (82.1)	35 (97.2)	264 (80.7%)	p<0.02
Father cooks	6 (2.1)	30 (83.3)	36 (11.0%)	p= 0.76
Grandmother cooks	61 (21.0)	5 (13.4)	66 (20.2%)	p= 0.22
High accessibility	188 (64.6)	31 (86.1)	219 (67.0%)	p<0.01
>4 hours/day of TV and videogames	121 (41.6)	13 (36.1)	134 (41.0%)	p=0.37
Risk of overweight	134 (59.0%)	53 (28.3%)	187 (57.5%)	p=0.24

[3] Personal characteristics and accessibility were divided into high and low according to the median.

With regards to personal and environmental correlates of VF consumption; a positive association was found between boy's BMI and higher VF consumption ($\chi^2 = 5.24$, $p<0.02$). This association was not observed in girls, nor was there an association between the BMI´s of both girls and boys and the hours spent viewing TV or playing videogames in children who reported eating 3 or more servings of vegetables and fruit per day.

There was no statistically significant association between knowledge, preference for fruits, or expectancy and higher VF intake. There was a higher VF intake when mothers were the ones that cooked at home most of the time ($\chi^2 = 5.24$, $p<0.02$) than when the father or grandmother did. There was a positive association ($\chi^2 = 6.699$; $p< 0.01$) between high VF accessibility and higher VF consumption in both girls and boys. The associations between self-efficacy and high VF intake ($\chi^2 = 3.937$; $p< 0.05$) and preferences for vegetables and vegetable consumption ($\chi^2 = 4.94$; $p< 0.03$) were statistically significant.

When running a stepwise logistic regression model with all the variables, accessibility (OR 3.38, 95% CI 1.26 - 9.0) and being a girl (OR 2.2, 95% CI 1.04 - 4.7) were the factors that correlated with a higher VF consumption.

Table 3. Parents personal and environmental characteristics[4] that correlate with vegetable and fruit consumption

	Vegetable and fruit intake			
Determinants	Lower 3 or less servings N= 40 (28.2%)	Higher 4 or more servings N=102 (71.8%)	Total n / N (142) n (%)	Statistical Significance
Personal				
High knowledge	8 (20.5%)	36 (37.5%	44 (32.6%)	p =0.05
High preferences for fruit	16 (41.0%)	48 (47.5%)	64 (45.7%)	p = 0.48
High preference for vegetables	12 (30.0%)	54 (52.9%)	66 (46.5%)	p = 0.014
High expectancy	13 (34.2%)	50 (50.5%)	63 (43.0%)	p = 0.08
High self-efficacy for fruit and vegetables	20 (54.1%)	48 (47.5%)	68 (49.3%)	p = 0.49
ENVIRONMENTAL				
High accessibility	11 (28.9%)	42 (42.4%)	53 (38.7%)	p = 0.14

[4] The personal characteristics and accessibility were divided into high and low according to the median. Total sample was 142; however, only results for positive variables are shown in the table.

Sample 2

Mean VF consumption reported by parents was 4.57±1.6 servings and the one reported for their children was 1.73±1.54. A positive association was found between knowledge (χ^2 =3.64, p< 0.05) and preference for vegetables (χ^2 =6.07, p<0.01) (Table 3). There was no statistically significant association between preferences for fruits, self-efficacy, accessibility or expectancy and higher VF intake. When running a stepwise logistic regression model with all the variables, knowledge (OR 1.63, 95% CI 1.23-2.17) was the variable that correlated with a higher VF consumption among parents. Parents' intake (OR 1.37, 95% CI 1.08-1.7) was the variable that correlated with a higher VF consumption among their children.

Discussion

Sample 1

The aim of this study was to identify the determinants of VF intake among Mexican children attending urban public schools in Mexico City. Through a multivariate model we determined that having high accessibility (OR 3.38, CI 1.26 to 9.0) to VF and being a girl (OR 2.2, CI 1.04 to 4.7) were the two factors that most influenced a higher (3 or more servings) intake of vegetables and fruit in this sample. We found that, in general, this population has a very low VF intake (1 serving per day on average) (Pomerleau et al., 2004) and that a large proportion of children do not consume VF at all (39%). This intake is very low when compared with the recommendations made by the World Cancer Research Fund (1997) (more than 5 servings/day or 400 g/day). This low VF intake is not particular to Mexican children; in Spain (Krebs-Smith, et al., 1996), one third of the children consume less than one serving a day; and in the United States the mean intake is 2.1 servings/day (Cullen et al., 2001). According to the National Institute of Public Health of Mexico (Rivera, 1999), the Mexican population consumes 2 servings/day on average. The results of this study (Figure 1) are similar to those of Sandvik et al. (2003) in that girls report a greater VF intake than boys (χ^2 = 6.022; p< 0.01).

Regarding the children's environmental variables related to the person in charge of cooking at home, our study shows that there was a higher VF consumption when the mother cooked at home than when any other family member did (χ^2 = 5.24; p<0.02). One explanation for this result might be that the mother is more concerned than others about providing the family with a "good meal" and, thus, tries to have better access to vegetables and fruit (Kratt et al., 2000).

Several studies (Cullen et al., 2003; Baxter and Schroder, 1997), have previously found high accessibility as the variable most associated with VF consumption. Blanchette et al., (2005) and Resnicow et al., (1997) found that availability, accessibility, and parents' example are the variables that most influence VF intake, and, therefore, intervention strategies to increase consumption should be based on these factors.

According to a focus group study with parents of similar children in the same schools (Pérez-Lizaur et al., unpublished data) parents believed that their children do not have the capacity and, in some instances, the interest to take part in the food preparation process, limiting their opportunities to be exposed to healthy eating habits. It would be interesting to explore how this belief affects children's accessibility to VF, and in which way could this barrier be overcome to benefit both the parents and their children. The parents in these focus groups mentioned that sometimes they find it difficult to prepare VF in a manner that is readily accessible to their children.

Self-efficacy refers to the confidence a person has in his or her capacity to perform the activities he or she wants to carry out (Bandura, 1986). Wolf and Campbell (1993) consider that self-efficacy is one determinant necessary for children to modify their behavior and increase VF consumption. Considering that self-efficacy is important for acquiring knowledge, it is interesting to note that in this study it was significantly associated (χ^2 = 3.937; $p< 0.05$) with a higher VF consumption in the bivariate analysis, even though it did not enter the stepwise logistic regression model. This could be due to the fact that χ^2 was borderline, and to the low consumption of VF among these children.

Preferences, knowledge, and expectancy were not associated with VF consumption in the bivariate analysis. Other studies have also shown no significant association between these variables and VF consumption (Cullen et al., 2000). In another study Dibsdall, et al (2003), suggests we need to focus on the motivation to eat fruits and vegetables, since no dietary improvement can be achieved if people do not recognize there is a problem.

VF consumption has been associated with BMI, and a low intake of these foods is associated with a greater prevalence of overweight in other populations (Biing and Mentzer, 2003). In our study, the greatest risk for overweight and obesity was found in boys (χ^2 = 4.826; $p< 0.03$), while in the Mexican National Nutrition Survey of 1999 (Hernández et al., 2003) the highest risk was among girls. The high risk for overweight and obesity in these children could be related to their parents' socioeconomic status (low to medium low). Several authors have suggested that a higher prevalence of obesity is observed when the parents have low educational attainment and low economic resources (Albala and Vio, 2000). In these cases, the availability of high-energy density foods and their low cost turns into a vicious cycle (Drewnowski and Darmon, 2005). It would be wise to review the incentives given to school stores and food support for families in need with special food stamps to purchase vegetables and fruits (Herman et al., 2006).

The children in our study spend, on average, 4 hours per day watching television and playing videogames; boys spend more time on these types of activities than girls ($\chi^2 = 4.665$; $p< 0.03$). Because boys spend more time performing sedentary activities than girls, they are at higher risk for overweight and obesity (Toussaint, 2000). Boynton-Jarrett and Thomas (2003) found in a study among adolescents that the more hours spent viewing television, the less was the VF consumption, even though a significant association could not be established.

Reed (2003) and Sturm and Datar (2005) suggest that in the last decades the world population has increased its weight and, at the same time, the price of VF has increased more rapidly than the price of other types of food and even more rapidly than the cost of living. The authors emphasize the need to modify the environment in order to produce an increase in VF consumption and decrease the overweight and obesity pandemic. At the same time, it is necessary to transfer new technologies that will increase the availability of sliced, ready-to-eat VF, eliminating the work of washing, cutting, slicing, and dicing them at home.

Sample 2

Through a multivariate model we determined that having knowledge of (χ^2 =3.64, p< 0.05) and a preference for vegetables (χ^2 =6.07, p<0.01), were the factors that correlated with a higher VF consumption among parents.

When running a stepwise logistic regression model with all the significant variables, knowledge (OR 1.63, CI 1.23-2.17) was the factor that most influenced a higher (4 or more servings) intake of VF among parents. Parents' intake (OR. 1.37, CI 1.09-1.7), was the factor that correlated with a higher VF (2 or more servings) consumption among their children.

We found that, in general parents reported a very high VF consumption (4 servings daily on average). We suspect this figure was an overestimate of their real VF consumption, a fact described by Bingham SA, *et. al.*, (1994). A similar conclusion was reached when reviewing data from the National Institute of Public Health of Mexico that report that the accurate VF daily consumption in Mexico is two servings (Rivera Dommarco et al., 2001).

In this study, knowledge referred to selecting, preparing and storing VF. In this sense, Larson NI, et al., (2006) report that adolescent children that participate in food preparation have a lower intake of fat and a higher FV consumption. Food skills intervention is likely to have a small but positive effect on food choice and confidence in food preparation. (Wrieden, WL. et al., (2007).

Other studies have found a positive association between knowledge of VF food guidelines and VF consumption (Campbell MK. et al., 2008). Wardle J. (2000) et al., have noted that knowledge is associated with healthy eating habits.

Even though the logistic regression analysis did not identify an association between preference for vegetables among parents, bivariate analysis did show it was associated with consumption among adults. Some authors have mentioned that preferences are directly related with consumption patterns (Cooke, 2007). It is believed that food preferences are established in the first years of life and so this is why health care providers should encourage VF consumption as one of the ways to reduce obesity among children (Lakakula AP et al., 2008).

We also found a positive association between FV consumption among parents and their children. Our results are in accordance with Pearson et al., (2008) who reports that consumption among parents is positively associated with consumption in their offspring. On the other hand, our results confirm the findings by Savage, et al., (2007) that state that the parents' eating behaviors modeled their children's eating choices. As mentioned in this study, "*parents select the composition of the family diet, serve as eating models that children tend to emulate and use eating practices to create the development of a culture of patterns and eating behaviors that are appropriate for their children*". Similar findings are reported by Cooke et al., (2003) and Brown (2004) who found that "fruit consumption among parents is a very strong predictor of fruit consumption among their children". Other studies have complemented these findings and have found a very strong link between knowledge of national guidelines and recommendations and vegetable intake. (De Bourdeaudhuij, I., 2008) asserts the role parents have among other variables in the consumption of VF in their children. In sum, the results put forth in our study indicate that the variables associated with VF consumption among children include accessibility, gender (being a girl) and parent's consumption of VF. The variable associated with the parent's VF consumption was knowledge (see Figure 1).

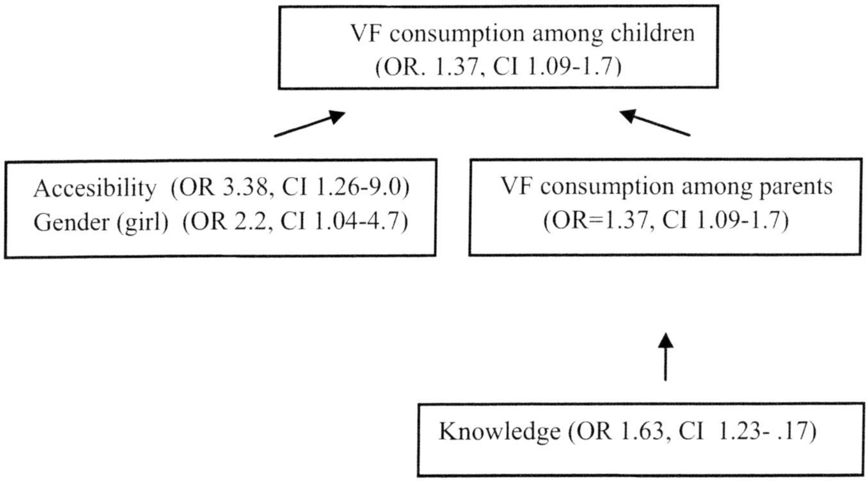

Figure 1. Determinants of vegetable and fruit consumption among children and their parents

Focus Groups

In order to enrich our study design and obtain qualitative data, we included a focus group that would assess the educational materials, and would help us design and evaluate the questionnaires (Vuckovic, N., Ritenaugh Ch A., 2000). Focus groups results were used to inform our study, adapt the data collection instruments and obtain relevant information on the subject.

The definition of a focus group is a meeting of people selected *a priori* to participate in a planned discussion with the aim of analyzing the degree of information, knowledge and experience each participant adds to the group via his or her opinions, perceptions, attitudes, beliefs and attempts at changing their behavior that in the context of a group creates a synergy effect. The main objective of a focus group organized with the children that participated in our study was to explore the variables associated with the consumption of fruits and vegetables among children in different primary school years, from the first to the third grade. The specific objectives for the focus group included in the first place, identify the relevant factors for children and adults in their VF consumption that would aid the study team in the design of the questionnaire. Some of the topics that were explored included perceptions regarding VF consumption, attitudes, motivations and barriers. The qualitative methodology employed allowed us to assess the level of language comprehension in the questionnaire as well as the cultural adequacy of the questions. One of the items read: *"do you understand the wording in the questionnaire and do you consider it culturally appropriate?"*

The results from the focus groups discussions were analyzed separately and then jointly. A report was drafted with the most relevant data. The main findings were classified into three main areas:

(a) Background. This section included which were their favorite fruits and vegetables and which were not liked, benefits associated with their consumption and sense of self efficacy.
(b) Daily food intake, explaining which were the meals and foods eaten at home and at school.
(c) Messages that are received both at home and at school on the subject of VF consumption.

Children

The three groups of children interviewed had a clear idea that eating fruits and vegetables is important for their growth and health. Nevertheless, it seemed as if knowledge alone was not sufficient enough to motivate them to consume VF more often or in higher quantities or in making them chose VF over other types of foods, especially highly processed ones. It is clear that choice is determined by other variables such as availability and ease of consuming a packaged snack where all you need to do is open the bag and eat it, does not require prior preparation, together with the pressure to consume these products that frequently are sold with some prize or toy. On the other hand, the reward for eating these foods is immediate and the benefits of eating a spinach salad are not too clear to a child, something that can constitute an important consumption barrier.

It would be interesting to explore mechanisms to build bridges between the abstract notion of "being healthy" and the time during break in which a child decides what to buy and eat. Children need more concrete examples of the ways in which they benefit from eating fruits and vegetables. A potential way of approaching children to healthy eating choices (in this case fruits and vegetables) would be for them to be in direct contact with them, to experiment with textures, colors, smells, colors, flavors. For children to grow, select, purchase, cook *etcetera,* in such a way that these food types would become meaningful to them. Natural curiosity that characterizes children could be another element that would draw them to consume fruits and vegetables more often.

For future research projects, it would be interesting to explore in small groups the experiences children have when exposed to different fruits and vegetables with questions that would invite them to describe their feelings when they eat an apple or when they get home and it smells of carrot soup. We speculate that the information derived from these types of questions could complement the data obtained in focus group discussions.

Another idea could involve working with children so they participate in food preparation, that is that they themselves could be in charge of preparing them and in this way have the chance to observe how they relate and interact with fruits and vegetables, the types of comments they make, the ideas that come up, the way in which they approach food (first I see it, then I feel it, I smell it, *etc.* I may even taste it). This could also become a way of empowering children to make healthy choices and ask for them or even participate in preparing foods they like.

It is interesting to note that in the three groups, children referred to vegetables in a positive manner. This stands in stark contrast with their parents testimonies that report their continuous worry that their children do not eat vegetables. This discrepancy could be further explored to try and explain why this is so and what are the positive variables that children associate with eating vegetables.

Finally it is important to mention that the information and role models provided by the school system regarding the consumption of fruits and vegetables is almost non existent. Children spend a great deal of time at school and yet the chance and opportunities they have to talk about, experience and consume fruits and vegetables is very limited. This aspect should be included in the Ministry of Education's teaching curricula.

Parents

Information from the focus groups carried out with parents was analyzed and the present report classifies findings into three main areas:

(a) Background. In this section worries and beliefs parents hold regarding their children´s eating patterns are included, especially their fruit and vegetable consumption.
(b) Daily eating, explains the types of dynamics that surround their children´s eating habits.
(c) Tools within the reach of parents that can help them increase the consumption of fruits and vegetables within the household.

In sum, in both focus groups, parents were engaged in their children´s health and the subject of eating patterns was an especially important item in the agenda. The concept that the consumption of fruits and vegetables is an important aspect of their children´s health was a recurrent subject yet at times they remarked that they often feel insecure about what types and quantities of FV they should feed them. The slogan "to grow up strong and healthy" or "to build their defenses or boost their immune system" did not seem to be enough information to convince their children of the importance of consuming vegetables when they do not wish to eat them.

Another topic that seemed to catch the parents´ attention and one in which they would benefit from, would be for them to be aware of their children´s general development and the changes in appetite, schedules and eating habits that children display throughout their different stages of growth. Clarifying doubts parents may have regarding the amount of fruits and vegetables that have to be consumed is directly related to a person´s overall health status and their age. The information parents have in these areas is minimal and they would like to be better informed. They welcomed the idea that both the school and teachers should play a more active role in this aspect of health and growth of their children. They even thought it valuable that the messages conveyed at home regarding health could be reinforced at school.

This is a promising research area to design policies and foster collaborations between the schools and parents.

Parents also discussed their interest in learning novel ways to prepare fruits and vegetables in order to increase the variety of foods they offer their families. Food presentation was one of the tools they identified as an effective way of getting their children to try vegetables that in "theory" children do not generally like. It would be interesting to further explore these curiosity sparked by parents and transmit it to their children.

Linked to this last point, it is worth noting that in general parents, mothers and fathers, assume their children do not have the ability and at times the interest in joining in the preparation of food and this aspect reduces the opportunities these offer to collaborate_and ultimately develop a more direct relationship with food. It would be interesting to explore the ways in which these beliefs have an influence in children´s disposition towards fruits and vegetables and the ways in these can be transformed to benefit both the parents and the children. During our focus group discussions parents mentioned that sometimes they find it difficult to prepare fruits and vegetables that are available all year round and that they would like for this to be possible. Maybe if snacks made from carrots or cucumbers were prepared with the help of children, the burden would be less and vegetables would be within the reach of children.

Finally, we suggest that the messages that are aimed at increasing the consumption of fruits and vegetables among children should be revised especially in the context of rewards and punishments and that alternative ways of relating to food in a pleasurable way may be found. In the case of fruits for example, the messages already used are more appealing, the language used is kinder and appeals to the senses (taste, touch). It would be important to capitalize on successful campaigns and invite them to continue pursuing them.

Possible limitations of this study are the validity of the diet assessment tool because of the age of the children and that it was a written self-administered procedure, may be not so appropriate for such young children. Also, the questions to measure knowledge and expectancy were insufficient to accurately measure these variables, although other authors (Traub, 1994) have also found this same problem with the Social Cognitive Theory; and the findings of this study cannot be generalized to other populations. In spite of these limitations, our study contributes to the field of nutrition by exploring Mexican children's and their parents′ eating habits by providing useful information to develop appropriate tools for nutrition education programs for Mexican children from low socioeconomic status.

Conclusions

Children's gender (being a girl) and the accessibility to VF were the variables that correlated with vegetable and fruit consumption in second- to fourth-grade elementary children from low socioeconomic groups in Mexico City. Home and school environments are fundamental for the children to increase VF consumption. It is also important to find creative ways to involve children in food preparation activities, to make them taste more VF so they increase their consumption. We found that VF consumption among parents is the variable more closely associated with consumption in children and that knowledge of VF is the one that better predicts consumption among parents. The results of our study convey a sense of urgency on the need to develop effective intervention strategies to promote VF consumption among children. Public health policies should target parents, teachers and children.

Acknowledgements

The authors wish to thank Paulina Chagoyán, Lidia Gil, Ivette Guzmán, Carolina Toledo, and Abigail Navarro for their valuable participation in data collection and field work. Roxana Valdés DSc and Alicia Beltrán MSc contributed with their expertise and were active participants during the standardization phase. The project was supported by the Universidad Iberoamericana and was part of Ana Bertha Pérez-Lizaur's Master's in Health Sciences at the State of Mexico Autonomous University (Universidad Autónoma del Estado de México). Martha Kaufer-Horwitz was the thesis director.

References

[1] Albala, C. and Vío, F. (2000) Obesidad y pobreza: un desafío pendiente en Chile. (Obesity and poverty: a pending challenge in Chile). In: *La obesidad en la pobreza: un nuevo reto para la salud pública.* eds. M. Peña and J. Bacallao, pp. 47-56. Washington, DC: OPS/OMS (OPS Publicación Científica No. 576).

[2] Comité de Niveles Socioeconómicos de la Asociación Mexicana de Agencias de Investigación de Mercados y Opinión Pública AC (AMAI) Mayo 2004. http://segmento.itam.mx/Administrador/Uploader/material/Niveles%20Socioeconomicos%20AMAI.PDF

[3] American Institute for Cancer Research/World Cancer Research Fund. (1997) *Food nutrition and the prevention of cancer: a global perspective.* Washington DC: AICR.

[4] Aranceta, J. and Serra Majem, L. (2001) Estructura General de las Guías Alimentarias para la Población Española. Decálogo para una dieta saludable. In: *SENC Guías alimentarias para la población española.* pp. 183-194. Madrid: SENC.

[5] Bandura, A. Social foundations of thought and action: a social cognitive theory. Englewood Cluffs, NJ. Prentice Hall 1986.

[6] Bandura, A. (2001) Self-efficacy: toward a unifying theory of behavioral change. *Psychol. Rev.* **84**, 191-215. Social Cognitive Theory: An agentic perspective. Annual Review of Psychology. 52, 1-26.

[7] Baranowski T, Perry Ch, Parcel G. (2002) How individuals, environments and health behavior interact. En Glanz K, Rimer B, Lewis F. Health Behavior and Health Education. Jossey-Bass.

[8] Baranowski, T., Lin, L.S., Wetter, D.W., Resnicow, K. and Eran, M.D. (1997) Theory as mediating variables: why aren't community interventions working as desired? *Ann. Epidemiol.* **7**, S89-S95.

[9] Baxter, I.A. and Schroder, M.J.A. (1997) Vegetable consumption among Scottish children: a review of the correlates and proposed strategies to overcome low consumption. *Br. Food J.* **99**, 380-387.

[10] Bazzano, L.A., He, J., Ogden, L.G., Loria, C.M., Vupputuri, S., Myers, M. and Whelton, P.K. (2002) Fruit and vegetable intake and risk of cardiovascular disease in US adults: the first National Health and Nutrition Examination Survey Epidemiologic Follow-up Study. *Am. J. Clin. Nutr.* **76**, 93-99.

[11] Biing-Hwan, W. and Mentzer, R. (2002) Higher fruit consumption linked with lower body mass index. *Food Rev.* **25**, 28-32

[12] Blanchette, l. and Brug, J. (2005) Correlates of fruit and vegetable consumption among 6-12-year-old children and effective interventions to increase consumption. *J. Hum. Nutr. Diet.* **18**, 431-443.

[13] Boynton-Jarrett, R. and Thomas, T. (2003) Impact of television viewing patterns on fruit and vegetable consumption among adolescents. *Pediatrics* **112**, 1321-1326.

[14] Branen, L.and Fletcher, J. (1999) Comparison of college students′ current eating habits and recollections of their childhood food practices. *J. Nutr. Educ.* **31**, 304-310.

[15] Bingham, SA., Gill, C., Welch, A., Day, K., Cassidy, A., Khaw, KT., Sneyd, MJ., Key, TJ., Roe, L., Day.and NE. (1994) Comparison of dietary assessment methods in nutritional epidemiology: weighed records v. 24 h recalls, food-frequency questionnaires and estimated-diet records. *Br J Nutr.***72**(4):619-43.

[16] Brown R, Ogden J.(2004) Children's eating attitudes and behaviour: a study of the modelling and control theories of parental influence. *Health Edu Res,* **19**(3):261-71.

[17] Campbell, MK:, Mc Lerran, Mc., Grievy, G., Feng, Z., Havas, S., Buller, D., Bereford, SA. and Nebeling, L.(2008) Mediation of adult fruit and vegetable consumption in the National 5 A Day for Better Health community studies. *Ann Behav Med.***35**(1):49-60.

[18] Carlton, T.B., Seymour J., Serdula, M., Kettel-Khan, L. and Rolls, B.J. (2004) What epidemiologic studies tell us about the relationship between fruit and vegetable consumption and body weight. *Nutr. Rev.* **62**, 365-374.

[19] Colgan, H. A., Floyd, S., Noone, E. J., Gibney, M. J. and Roche, H. M. (2004) Increased intake of fruit and vegetables and a low-fat diet, with and without low-fat plant sterol-enriched spread consumption: effects on plasma lipoprotein and carotenoid metabolism . *Journal of Human Nutrition and Dietetics* **17** (6), 561-569.

[20] Cooke, L., Wardle, J. and Gibson, EL. (2003) Relationship between parental report of food neophobia and everyday food consumption in 2-6 year old children. *Appetite.*;**41**(2):205-6.

[21] Cooke L. (2007) The importance of exposure for healthy eating in childhood: a review. *J Hum Nutr Diet.* **20**(4):294-301.

[22] Cullen, K.W., Baranowski, T., Owens, E., Marsh, T., Rittenberry, L. and de Moor, C. (2003) Availability, accessibility, and preferences for fruit, 100% fruit juice, and vegetables influence children's dietary behavior. *Health Educ. Behav.* **30**, 615-626.

[23] Cullen, K.W., Baranowski, T., Rittenberry, L., Cosart, C., Hebert, D. and de Moor, C. (2001) Child-reported family and peer influences on fruit, juice and vegetable consumption: reliability and validity of measures. *Health Educ. Res.* **16**, 187-200.

[24] Cullen, K.W., Baranowski, T., Rittenberry, L. and Olvera, N. (2000) Social-environmental influences on children's diets: results from focus groups with African-, Euro-, and Mexican-American children and their parents. *Health Educ. Res.* **15**, 581-590.

[25] De Bourdeaudhuij., te Velde, S., Brug, J., Due, J., Wind, M., Sandvik, C., Maes, L., Wolf, A., Perez-Rodrigo, C., Yngbe, A., Thorsdottir, L., Rasmussen, M., Elmadfa, I., Franchini, B. and Kleep, KL. (2008) Personal, social and environmental predictors of daily fruit and vegetable intake in 11-year-old children in nine European countries. *Eur J Clin Nutr*. 62(7):834- 41.

[26] De Irala-Estevez, J., Groth, M., Johansson, L., Oltersdorf, U., Prattala, R. and Martinez-Gonzalez, M.A. (2000) A systematic review of socioeconomic differences in food habits in Europe: consumption of fruit and vegetables. *European J. Clin. Nutr.* **54**, 706-714.

[27] Dibsdall, L.A., Lambert, N., Bobbin, R.F. and Frewer, L.J. (2003) Low-income consumers'attitudes and behaviour towards access, availability and motivation to eat fruit and vegetables. *Public Health Nutr.* **6**,159-168.

[28] Drewnowski, A. and Darmon, N. (2005) The economics of obesity: dietary energy density and energy cost. *Am. J. Clin. Nutr.* **82**, 265S-273S.

[29] Drewnowski, A. and Barrat-Fornell, A. (2003) Do healthier diets cost more? *Nutr. Today* **39**, 161-168.

[30] Elfhag, K. and Rasmussen, F. (2008) Food consumption, eating behaviour and self-esteem among single v. married and cohabiting mothers and their 12-year-old children. *Public Health Nutr.*11(9):934-9.

[31] EURO DIET (2001) Nutrition and Diet for Healthy Lifestyles in Europe: the EURODIET Evidence. Public Health Nutrition Vol 4. 2(A) and 2(B).

[32] The European Food Information Council (EUFIC) http://www.eufic.org/sp/fodd/pag/food45/food451.htm, accessed on 10 November 2004.

[33] Glanz, K., Lewis, F.M. and Rimer, B. eds. (1997) *Health behavior and health education: theory, research and practice.* Second Edition. San Francisco: Jossey-Bass, Inc.

[34] Gunde, R. (2002). School Children in the Developing World: Health, Nutrition and School Performance http://www.international.ucla.edu/article.asp?parentid=8943

[35] Hayes, D.P. (2005) The protective role of fruits and vegetables against radiation-induced cancer. *Nutr. Rev.* **63**, 303-311.

[36] Herman, D. and Harrison, G. (2006) Choices made by low-income women provided with an economic supplement for fresh fruit and vegetable purchase. *J. Am. Diet. Assoc.* **106**, 740-744.

[37] Hernández, B., Cuevas-Nasu, L., Shamah-Levy, T. and Rivera, J. (1999) Factores asociados con sobrepeso y obesidad en niños mexicanos de edad escolar: resultados de la Encuesta Nacional de Nutrición, 1999.

[38] Klepp, K. I. , Pérez-Rodrigo' C. , De Bourdeaudhuij, I., Pernille Due, P. , Elmadfa, I., et al (2005) Promoting fruit and vegetable consumption among European schoolchildren:

Rationale, conceptualization and design of the Pro Children Project. *Annals of Nutrition and Metabolism* **49**:212-220

[39] Kratt, P., Reynolds, K. and Shewchuk, R. (2000) The role of availability as a moderator of family fruit and vegetable consumption. *Health Educ. Behav.* **27**, 471-482.

[40] Krebs-Smith, S.M., Cook, A., Subar, A.F., Cleveland, L., Friday, J. and Kahle, L.L. (1996) Fruit and vegetable intakes of children and adolescents in the United States. *Arch. Pediatr. Adolesc. Med.* **150**, 81-86.

[41] Lakkakula, AP., Zanovec, M., Silverman, L., Murphy, E. and Tuuri, G. (2008) Black children with high preferences for fruits and vegetables are at less risk of being at risk of overweight or overweight. *J Am Diet Assoc.***108**(11):1912-5.

[42] Larson NI, Neumark-Sztainer DR, Harnack LJ, Wall MM, Story MT, Eisenberg ME. (2008) Fruit and vegetable intake correlates during the transition to young adulthood. *Am J Prev Med.* **35**(1):33-37.

[43] Liu, S., Manson, J.E., Lee, I-M., Cole, S.R., Hennekens, C.H., Willett, W.C. and Buring, J.E. (2000) Fruit and vegetable intake and risk of cardiovascular disease: the Women´s Health Study. *Am. J. Clin. Nutr.* **72**, 922-928.

[44] Lohman, T., Roche, A. and Martorell, R. (1988) *Anthropometric standardization reference manual*. Champaign, Illinois: Human Kinetics Books.

[45] Must, A., Dallal, G.E. and Dietz, W.H. (1991) Reference data for obesity: 85th and 95th percentiles of body mass index (wt/ht^2) and triceps skinfold thickness. *Am. J. Clin. Nutr.* **53**, 839-846.

[46] National Center for Health Statistics (NCHS). 2000 CDC Growth Charts: United States. http://www.cdc.gov/growthcharts.

[47] Norma Oficial Mexicana (2004) NOM-043 SSA2–2004, Servicios Básicos de Salud, Promoción y Educación para la Salud en Materia Alimentaria. Criterios para Brindar Orientación. Official Mexican Standard NOM-043-SSA2-2004, to provide Nutrition Education to the Public.

[48] Perarson, N., Biddle, SJ. and Gorely, T. (2008) Family correlates of fruit and vegetable consumption in children and adolescents: a systematic review. *Public Health Nutr.* 18:1-17.

[49] Pérez, R.C., Aranceta, J., Brug, H. and Wind, M. (2004) Estrategias educativas para la promoción del consumo de frutas y verduras en el medio escolar: proyecto pro children. *Arch. Latinoam. de Nutr.* **54**, S14-S19.

[50] Pérez-Lizaur AB, Kaufer-Horwitz M, Plazas M. (2008) Environmental and personal correlates of fruit and vegetable consumption in low income, urban Mexican children. J Hum Nut Diet **21**, 63-71.

[51] Pomerleau, J., Lock, K., McKee, M., Altmann, D. (2004) The Challenge of Measuring Global Fruit and Vegetable Intake. J. Nutr. **134**,1175-1180,

[52] Prieto, L. and Badia, X. (2001) Cuestionarios de salud: concepto y metodología. *Atención Primaria* **28**, 201-209.

[53] Reed, A. (2003) Commentary: Farley T, Cohen D. Prescription for a healthy nation. *J. Am. Med. Assoc.* **293**, 2800.

[54] Resnicow, K., Davis-Hearn, M., Smith, M., Baranowski, T., Lin, L.S., Baranowski, J., Doyle, C. and Wang, D.T. (1997) Social-cognitive predictors of fruit and vegetable intake in children. *Health Psychol.* **16**, 272-276.

[55] Riboli, E. and Norat, T. (2003) Epidemiologic evidence of the protective effect of fruit and vegetables on cancer risk. *Am. J. Clin. Nutr.* **78**, 559S-569S.

[56] Rivera Dommarco, J., Shamah Levy, T., Villalpando Hernández, S., González de Cossío, T., Hernández Prado, B. and Sepúlveda, J. (2001) Encuesta Nacional de Nutrición 1999. Estado nutricio de niños y mujeres en México. Cuernavaca Morelos, México. Instituto Nacional de Salud Pública.

[57] Rolls, B.J., Ello-Martin, J.A. and Carlton, T.B. (2004) What can intervention studies tell us about the relationship between fruit and vegetable consumption and weight management? *Nutr. Rev.* **62**, 1-17.

[58] Sandvik, C., De Bourdeaudhuij, I., Due, P., Brug, J., Wind, M., Bere, E., Pérez-Rodrigo, C., Wolf, A., Elmadfa, I., Thórsdóttir, I., Vaz de Almeida. M.D., Yngve, A. and Klepp, K-I. (2005) Personal, social and environmental factors regarding fruit and vegetable intake among schoolchildren in nine European countries. *Ann. Nutr. Metab.* **49**, 255–266.

[59] Savage JS, Fisher JO, Birch LL. (2007) Parental influence on eating behavior: conception to adolescence. *J Law Med Ethics.* **35**(1):22-34.

[60] Scaglioni S, Salvioni M, Galimberti C. (2008) Influence of parental attitudes in the development of children eating behaviour. *Br J Nutr.* **99** Suppl 1:S22-5.

[61] Sylvestre MP, O'Loughlin J. (2007) Gray Donald K, Hanley J, Paradis G. Association between fruit and vegetable consumption in mothers and children in low-income, urban neighborhoods. *Health Educ Behav.* **34**(5):723-34.

[62] Satia, J. A., Kristal, A.R., Patterson, R.E., Neuhouser, M.L. (2002) Psychosocial factors and dietary habits associated with vegetable consumption. *Nutrition.* **18**, 247-254.

[63] Sichieri, R. (2002) Dietary patterns and their associations with obesity in the Brazilian city of Rio de Janeiro. *Obes. Res.* **10**, 42-48.

[64] Streiner, D. and Norman, G. (2003) *Health measurement scales: a practical guide to their development and use.* 3rd edn. New York: Oxford University Press.

[65] Sturm, R. and Datar, A. (2005) Body mass index in elementary school children, metropolitan area food prices and food outlet density. *Public Health* **119**, 1059-1068.

[66] Traub,R.E. (1994) Reliability for the Social Sciences, Theory and Applications. Thousan Oak, Calif: Sage Pub.

[67] Toussaint, M.G. (2000) Patrones de dieta y actividad física en la patogénesis de la obesidad en el escolar urbano. *Bol. Méd. Hosp. Infant. Méx.* **57**, 650-662.

[68] Voorrips, L.E., Goldbohm, R.A., van Poppel, G., Sturmans, F., Hermus, R.J.J. and van den Brandt, P.A. (2000) Vegetable and fruit consumption and risks of colon and rectal cancer in a prospective cohort study the Netherlands cohort study on diet and cancer. *Am. J. Epidemol.* **152**, 1081-1092.

[69] Wardle, J., Parmenter, K. and Waller, J.Nutrition (2000) knowledge and food intake. *Appetite.* **34**(3):269-75.

[70] Wolfe, W.S. and Campbell, C.C. (1993) Food pattern, diet quality, and related characteristics of schoolchildren in New York State. *J. Am. Diet Assoc.* **93**, 1280-1284.

[71] World Cancer Research Fund (1997). Food, Nutrition and the Prevention of Cancer: a global perspective. Cap 8. Diet and Health Recommendations for the Prevention of Cancer.

[72] World Health Organization. (2003) Integrated prevention of noncommunicable diseases. Draft global strategy on diet, physical activity and health. Executive Board. 113th Session WHO.

[73] Yngve, A., Wolf, A., Poortvliet, E., Elmadfa, I., Brug, J., Ehrenblad, B., Franchini, B., Haraldsdottir, J., Krolner, R., Maes, L., Perez-Rodrigo, C., Sjostrom, M., Thorsdottir, I. and Klepp, K.I. (2005) Fruit and vegetable intake in a sample of 11-year-old children in 9 European countries: The Pro Children Cross-sectional Survey. *Ann. Nutr. Metab.* **49**, 236-245.

In: Fruit and Vegetable Consumption and Health
Editors: Anton Papareschi and Harvey Eppolito
ISBN: 978-1-60741-596-1

Chapter 4

Vegetable Intake as Preventive Measure against Type 2 Diabetes and Cancer

***Nurgül Fitzgerald*[a] *and Niyati Parekh*[b]**
[a]Department of Nutritional Sciences, Rutgers, The State University of New Jersey
[b]Department of Nutrition, Food Studies and Public Health, New York University

Abstract

Type 2 diabetes and cancer are among the leading causes of death in the United States, and the etiology of both diseases is linked to dietary intake. This chapter includes an overview of the studies that examined the relationships between vegetable consumption, and type 2 diabetes and various cancers. Potential mechanisms of action that might be underlying the associations between vegetable intake and type 2 diabetes or cancer risk have also been discussed. Briefly, several studies point out the probable protective influence of vegetable intake against type 2 diabetes and various cancers. However, not all studies agree on this potential protective effect. Some of this disagreement might be coming from the methodological differences between the studies. It is possible that various nutrients and non-nutrient components in vegetables and other foods might be exerting protective effects cumulatively. Additionally, diets high in vegetables might be replacing less healthful intake patterns or might be related to diabetes and cancer via complex relationships with other lifestyle characteristics and disease risk factors (e.g., obesity). Considering that studies do not indicate an increased risk of type 2 diabetes or cancer with higher non-starchy vegetable consumption, aiming for diets that are higher in non-starchy vegetables seem to be a valuable nutrition and public health strategy.

Introduction

Diabetes mellitus and cancer affect millions of people, and they are among the leading causes of death in the United States of America (US) [1, 2]. According to the 2007 estimates, about 23.6 million people or 7.8% of the population in the US have diabetes [3]. It is estimated that about 180 million people worldwide have diabetes, and this number is expected to double by year 2030 [4]. Similarly, the number of cancer survivors, defined as individuals having a cancer diagnosis regardless of course of the illness, is projected to double by 2050 [5].

Although type 2 diabetes and cancer have genetic causes, other – modifiable – factors, such as obesity, physical activity, and food intake, influence the pathophysiology of both diseases [6, 7]. Among the various dietary factors, existing literature points to the potential protective roles of plant foods, such as fruits, vegetables, legumes, and whole grains against type 2 diabetes and cancer, and the literature regarding vegetable intake in relationship to these chronic diseases will be reviewed in this chapter.

Before summarizing the published literature, it might be helpful to explain some of the relevant methodological terminology. Most of the results included in this chapter originate from epidemiologic studies, which may involve cross-sectional (i.e., data collection at one time point only), case-control (selection and comparison of groups with and without the disease), cohort or prospective (follow-up of individuals longitudinally) designs, and also meta-analyses, where results of several studies of the similar designs are analyzed together to obtain summary risk estimates. Disease risk estimates in these studies may be expressed as relative risk (RR), hazard ratio (HR), or odds ratio (OR) with their corresponding 95% confidence interval (CI) or p-values. Generally, risk estimate values that are less than one represent protective associations between vegetable consumption and disease (diabetes or cancer), whereas estimates greater than one represent detrimental associations. Confidence intervals that include the value of one represent the lack of statistically significant association between the food intake and disease.

Following sections will present an overview of the published literature about the associations between vegetable intake and risk for type 2 diabetes and various cancers.

I. Vegetable Intake and Type 2 Diabetes: Evidence From The Literature

Diabetes mellitus is defined as a group of metabolic diseases characterized by increased levels of plasma glucose (hyperglycemia) resulting from the defects in insulin secretion in the pancreas, insulin action at various tissues, or both. Although there are other subcategories of diabetes mellitus, type 2 diabetes constitutes about 90-95% of all diabetes cases [8]. In addition to the insulin resistance and hyperglycemia, low-grade inflammation, changes in endothelial function, hypertension, and dyslipidemia are common and contribute to the long-term complications of this disease. Heart attack, stroke, blindness, lower extremity amputations, and kidney failure are examples of long-term and often life-threatening complications of diabetes mellitus [9].

Several susceptibility genes for type 2 diabetes have been identified [10], and certain racial/ethnic groups (e.g., Hispanics/Latinos, Native Americans, Asian/Pacific Islanders, etc.) appear to have higher rates of type 2 diabetes [3], but environmental factors are also known to influence type 2 diabetes etiology. Obesity, and lifestyle characteristics such as physical inactivity and certain dietary intake patterns are among these modifiable risk factors [6, 11].

Examining the associations between dietary intake and risk of chronic disease can involve various approaches such as looking at the intakes of individual or combinations of food groups (e.g., fruits, vegetables, or fruits and vegetables), individual foods, or nutrients (e.g., vitamins or minerals). Because it is extremely difficult in controlled experimental studies or long-term randomized clinical trials to retain a large number of individuals on a particular diet with appropriate control and accurate measurement of all dietary components, researchers sometimes utilize statistical techniques to determine the overall intake patterns. Using such an approach (factor analysis) in a large prospective study among male health professionals in the US, Van Dam et al. determined a "prudent" and a "western" dietary intake pattern in relationship to type 2 diabetes risk [12]. The prudent dietary intake pattern, which was characterized by greater intakes of fruits and vegetables (excluding potatoes) alongside legumes, poultry, fish, and whole grains, showed a tendency toward a protective effect against type 2 diabetes (OR:0.84, 95% CI:0.70-1.00) after adjusting for a wide range of other likely risk factors. Individuals, who consumed the highest (versus lowest) level of prudent diet were 16% less likely to have type 2 diabetes. The western dietary pattern was characterized by greater intakes of red or processed meats, fried potatoes, refined grains, high-fat dairy, sweets and desserts. Interestingly, the positive association between incidence of type 2 diabetes and western dietary intake pattern was considerably stronger (OR:1.59, 95% CI:1.32-1.93); individuals at the highest level of western dietary intake pattern were about 59% more likely to have type 2 diabetes compared to those who had the lowest intake levels for this diet type. These results suggest that although a healthier dietary intake pattern, including higher intake of vegetables, might be protective against type 2 diabetes, the potential detrimental influence of a less healthy intake pattern may have a greater influence on the risk for type 2 diabetes.

Other studies have examined the potential relationship of individual food groups and type 2 diabetes. Ford and Mokdad [13] examined these associations for fruit and vegetable intake in the prospective National Health and Nutrition Examination Survey (NHANES) I Epidemiologic Follow-up Study, which included about 20-year follow-up data from 9,665 adults, who were 25-74 years of age at the baseline. Ford and Mokdad reported that consuming five or more fruits and vegetables per day was related to a lower risk of diabetes among women after adjusting for a variety factors, such as age, race/ethnicity, cigarette smoking, hypertension, serum cholesterol levels, body mass index (BMI), physical activity, and alcohol intake [13]. However, further adjustment for participants' education level attenuated these associations, which points out the complex associations of diet, other lifestyle or personal characteristics, and health outcomes.

Studies outside the US also suggest a likely protective effect agaist diabetes with greater vegetable consumption. A 23-year follow-up of a prospective study among 4,034 adults (aged 40-69 years) in Finland indicated that a dietary pattern characterized by greater intakes of fruits and vegetables was related to a 28% lower risk of type 2 diabetes (RR:0.72, 95% CI:0.53-0.98) [14]. Among the types of vegetables, green vegetable intake showed the strongest association after adjusting for age, gender, BMI, energy intake, smoking, family history of diabetes, and geographic area. The highest (versus the lowest) quartile of green vegetable intake was related to a 31% less risk (RR:0.69, 95% CI:0.50-0.93) of having type 2 diabetes. Interestingly, consumption of potatoes was more closely associated with the intakes of red meat, whole milk, and butter rather than fruits and vegetables [15].

A cross-sectional study among Native Canadians even suggested a negative association between vegetable consumption and an earlier metabolic disturbance leading to diabetes. In this study, vegetable intake (third quartile vs. first quartile) was negatively related to having diabetes, or impaired glucose tolerance, which is a phase that precedes overt type 2 diabetes (OR:0.51, 95% CI:0.28-0.92). Although vegetable intake was not related to obesity in this study, it is not known whether the detected association was independent of other diabetes risk factors since the results were only adjusted for age and gender [16]. Similarly, results from the 20-year follow-up of the prospective Seven Countries Study also indicated an inverse association between plasma glucose levels (during a glucose tolerance test) and vegetable and legume intake after adjusting for age, baseline measures, cohort, BMI, and energy intake [17]. Because vegetables and legumes were combined into one group in this study, it is not clear whether detected associations would differ if the two food groups were examined separately.

More detailed information about the specific types of vegetables and risk of type 2 diabetes comes from a prospective study among women in China. This study indicated that intakes of several types of vegetables (cruciferous, green/leafy, yellow, allium, tomatoes, or other vegetables) were negatively related to type 2 diabetes risk after adjusting for other likely confounders (age, energy, meat and alcohol intakes, BMI, physical activity, socioeconomic status, etc.) [18]. The findings from the cross-sectional European Prospective Investigation into Cancer (EPIC-Norfolk) study among adults without diabetes are in agreement with the results of the Chinese study: individuals who never or seldom consumed green leafy vegetables had higher blood glucose levels in comparison to those who consumed these vegetables five or more times per week. This association was independent of potential influences of dietary fiber, vitamin C, and energy intakes, or other likely confounders, such as BMI, age, gender, physical activity, alcohol intake or cigarette smoking [19]. Although this was a cross-sectional study, exclusion of individuals with diabetes strengthens the study findings because individuals who already have type 2 diabetes might have changed their dietary intake because of their disease.

Although aforementioned studies tend to support a protective effect of greater vegetable consumption probably in combination with other healthful dietary patterns, it is not clear what proportions of these associations involve direct versus indirect relationships between vegetable intake and risk for type 2 diabetes. As mentioned earlier, Ford and Mokdad [13] reported in a large prospective study that the association between fruit and vegetable intake and diabetes was affected by education level of the participants. Liu et al. [20] reported another likely effect modification by overweight status in an analysis of the prospective Women's Health Study. In this study, dark yellow or green leafy vegetable intakes were related to a decreased risk of type 2 diabetes only among overweight women. Similarly, a cross-sectional study among 1,053 adults, aged 40-64 years, indicated that vegetable consumption was related to a lower likelihood of having type 2 diabetes (OR:0.16, 95% CI:0.04-0.81) after adjusting for age, family history of diabetes, and gender, but this association was attenuated after controlling for BMI [21]. The potential association between fruit and vegetable intake and weight status is further supported by a 12-year follow up of the prospective Nurses' Health Study, which included over 74,000 female registered nurses. This study indicated that highest (fifth quintile) increase in fruit and vegetable intake over the years was related to a 16% lower likelihood of becoming obese after adjusting for a wide range of factors such as age, physical activity, smoking, energy, caffeine, alcohol, and macronutrient intakes (OR:0.84, 95% CI:0.75-0.93) [22]. Overall, these studies suggest that there might be direct and indirect associations between vegetable intake and type 2 diabetes.

Despite these findings, which generally indicate protective associations between type 2 diabetes and diets involving higher intake levels of vegetables, the research results on this topic are not unanimous. In a recent meta-analysis of five cohort studies, Hamer and Chida [23] did not find a significant association between consuming three servings or more (and alternatively, five servings or more) vegetables per day and incidence of type 2 diabetes. However, there was an inverse association between type 2 diabetes incidence and antioxidant intake. Because fruits and vegetables are the likely dietary sources of antioxidants, vegetables might be exerting a protective effect through their antioxidant properties, and this potential mechanism will be reviewed further in the next section.

Additionally, it is not clear whether the potential protective effect of vegetable consumption against type 2 diabetes is stemming from vegetables alone, or in concert with the intake of variety of other healthful foods (e.g., fruits, legumes, whole grains), lower intake of less healthful foods, or a combination of all. The number of studies that examined the intakes of various vegetables while controlling for all other likely risk factors is still limited, and future research is needed. The following section will provide an overview of the potential mechanisms that may be underlying the associations between vegetable intake and type 2 diabetes.

II. Vegetable Consumption and Potential Protective Mechanisms Against Type 2 Diabetes

Underlying mechanisms of action for the potential protective effect of vegetable consumption against type 2 diabetes can be via the antioxidant or other functions of micronutrients (i.e., vitamins and minerals) or phytochemicals, or through the fiber content. It is also possible that diets high in vegetables may be protective against type 2 diabetes by replacing less healthful dietary intake patterns (e.g., those with higher energy density) that may lead to weight gain and obesity, which is a major risk factor for this disease.

Vegetables might be protective against type 2 diabetes through the antioxidant properties of their nutrient and phytochemical content. Phytochemicals (e.g., flavonoids, isoflavones, glucosinolates, organosulphur compounds, saponins, and phytosterols) are non-nutrient food components with important biologic properties. Antioxidants, such as flavonoids, carotenoids, and vitamins C and E in vegetables may prevent oxidative stress [24, 25], especially in the pancreatic beta-cells that produce insulin. A meta-analysis of five cohort studies provides some support for this potential mechanism since no significant association was detected between vegetable intake and type 2 diabetes incidence, but there was a significant inverse relationship between antioxidant intake and type 2 diabetes. Further, this effect was mostly coming from vitamin E and total carotenoids [23]. These findings should not be taken as convincing evidence to begin recommending vitamin supplementation as a protection against diabetes because these effects were detected for intake levels that would most likely be met by regular food intake. Additionally, other studies [26, 27] that examined the associations between type 2 diabetes and vitamin E or carotenoid supplements do not provide evidence of additional protective effect with supplementation. Therefore, it is possible that several antioxidants from various vegetables and other foods might be exerting a protective effect synergistically.

Phytochemicals' anti-inflammatory or other protective functions may also be underlying the associations between vegetable intake and type 2 diabetes. Inflammatory response is known to play a role in the progression of insulin resistance and type 2 diabetes [24] leading to cardiovascular complications of this disease. Hence, phytochemicals such as polyphenols from vegetables may be slowing down the progress of type 2 diabetes by preventing the likely vascular complications through anti-inflammatory or vasorelaxant effects, which would help protect vascular wall from cell proliferation. Additionally, another group of phytochemicals, flavonoids, have been reported to increase enzyme activity that counteracts the sorbitol accumulation through the polyol reductase pathway, that often leads to neuropathy, nephropathy, and retinopathy (e.g., cataracts, blindness), which are common long-term complications of type 2 diabetes [24].

Plant polyphenols may also have direct influence on the blood glucose levels through their effects on digestion and absorption of nutrients. Polyphenols have been reported to inhibit enzymatic activities of alpha-amylase and sucrase, which are normally needed for the digestion of carbohydrates. Additionally, polyphenols (e.g., saponins, isoflavones, and tannic acid) have been reported to delay the gastric emptying and/or decrease the intestinal transport of glucose, and as a result, help regulate blood glucose levels after a meal [24].

Determining the individual effects of phytochemicals is a challenge because of the existence of hundreds of these compounds in various foods. Further complicating the issue is the fact that some of the existing literature have examined vegetables and fruits as a single food group. Because fruits are also rich in several phytochemicals, it is not known how much of the detected associations truly reflect the contribution of vegetables alone. For example, chlorogenic acid in wild berries and coffee has been indicated to decrease the transport of glucose from proximal duodenum; resveratrol has been reported to have an anti-inflammatory effect and also increase the glucose transporter GLUT-4 expression in the muscle tissue; and anthocyanins from berries have been reported to decrease inflammatory response, oxidative damage, and glucose absorption [24]. Further research is needed to clarify these associations.

In addition to the phytochemicals, nutrients such as vitamins and minerals found in vegetables may be contributing to the potential protective effects of vegetables. Potassium, which is found in higher amounts in plant-based diets, has been reported to lower blood pressure, and this may consequentially protect against vascular damage that is associated with type 2 diabetes. Similarly, folate intake is inversely related to plasma homocysteine levels, which is related to an increased risk for cardiovascular disease [28], and green leafy vegetables are a rich source of folate. Magnesium could be another mineral with a protective role against type 2 diabetes because it plays key roles in the carbohydrate metabolism, and a meta-analysis of seven cohort studies showed an inverse association between magnesium intake and type 2 diabetes [29]. However, others reported a threshold effect, where protective influence was confined to individuals with some level of magnesium deficiency [30].

In addition to the mechanisms related to phytochemicals, vitamins, and minerals, another potential protective mechanism can be via the fiber content of vegetables. Dietary fiber may be protective against type 2 diabetes through its effects on inflammation, digestion and absorption of other carbohydrates, gastric emptying, intestinal microbial flora, satiety, or weight status [31]. Although plant-based or high-fiber diets may also supply more minerals such as magnesium, the protective association between high-fiber diets and type 2 diabetes seem to be independent of the magnesium intake [32].

Similar to the phytochemicals, high-fiber diets have been reported to be associated with a decrease in the inflammatory response [31], and this may be protective against the vascular damage and complications of type 2 diabetes.

Fruits and vegetables mostly provide soluble fiber which has been reported to delay gastric emptying and decrease glucose absorption in the intestines, and this process results in a more favorable glucose response after consuming a meal [24, 28]. Greater dietary fiber intake, in general, has also been reported to be associated with lower fasting insulin levels [33]. Additionally, soluble fiber is highly fermentable by the bacteria in the colon. The product of this fermentation is the short-chain fatty acids, which have been linked to improved blood lipid levels and decreased glucose production in the liver [31].

High fiber intake through vegetables might also be contributing to a protective effect against type 2 diabetes by producing a greater level of satiation and decreased feeling of hunger after meals [31]. This effect can lead to a lower level of energy intake and less likelihood of obesity in the long-term. Several published studies suggest that diets that are characterized by a higher intake of fruits and vegetables are likely to have a lower energy density, and such higher fiber diets are inversely related to overweight or obesity [22, 33-35]. Therefore, the relationship between vegetable intake and type 2 diabetes can be mediated or modified through obesity, which is a major diabetes risk factor. Although many of the studies control for obesity when examining the associations between type 2 diabetes and vegetable intake, there may still be unmeasured influence stemming from weight status.

In summary, many studies suggest the presence of protective associations between type 2 diabetes and higher consumption of vegetables, or a combination of vegetables, fruits, and other higher fiber foods (e.g., legumes, whole grains). Although several potentially protective mechanisms of action (e.g., nutrients' and phytochemicals' anti-inflammatory, vasorelaxant, or antioxidant properties, effects of high-fiber diets on digestion, nutrient absorption, and glucose metabolism, insulin sensitivity, or obesity) have been reported, specific role and magnitude of these potential effects still need clarification.

There also exist studies that do not show a statistically significant relationship between vegetable consumption and risk for type 2 diabetes. One of the likely reasons for these results can be the possibility that several macro and micronutrients and other components such as phytochemicals in vegetables and other foods might be exerting their protective effects in a cumulative or synergistic fashion [36]. Hence, the individual influence of each nutrient may be too small to show an independent protective effect. Evidence from the literature provides some support for this probability. For example, the literature indicated a negative association between serum carotenoids and serum insulin levels [37], and a protective association between type 2 diabetes and yellow vegetables [18], which are a major source of carotenoids. However, a randomized clinical trial of beta-carotene supplementation did not show any protective effect against type 2 diabetes in a large study in the US [26].

Accurately determining vegetable or any other food intake also has its challenges and could potentially influence the study results. For example, underreporting of less healthful foods and overreporting of more healthful foods (e.g. fruits and vegetables) especially among obese individuals can affect the study findings. In addition, higher prevalence of obesity and over-consumption of various nutrients in typical western diets may make it difficult to detect any potential protective effects of individual nutrients, especially those that might show their protective effects only among individuals with a certain degree of nutrient deficiency (i.e. threshold effect).

Examining only vegetable or any other single food group intake might also be an unrealistically narrow perspective when looking into the potential influence of diet on chronic disease risk. It is possible that individuals, who have lower consumption levels for vegetables, might be replacing vegetables with less healthful foods with greater energy and lower nutrient density. As a result, examining only vegetables may not reflect the true disease risk without looking into the intakes of other foods. Hence, it is not known whether the intake level of vegetables is an adequate indicator for all the other changes in the diet.

Furthermore, some studies suggest that the effect of vegetable consumption might be modified by other factors, such as education level or obesity status. Although higher consumption of vegetables seem to be protective against type 2 diabetes, vegetable intake is only one of the characteristics of an overall healthier lifestyle, which must be taken into account when examining the associations between dietary intake and diabetes risk.

III. Vegetable Consumption and Cancer

Cancer is a disease of altered gene expression, and it is caused by accumulation of insults to the DNA, which makes up the genetic material. Cancer manifests as uncontrolled cell growth because of a loss in control of the normal growth cycle and replication process. Cancer cells may evade apoptosis and growth inhibitory signals, which results in growth signal autonomy [38]. Cancer cells are capable of invading and surviving in other tissues, causing metastasis, and potentially leading to death [38]. Most cancers develop to a clinically important stage several years after DNA damage. A major cause of DNA damage is oxidative stress [39]. Reactive oxidative species, which are products of normal metabolisms [40], are capable of attacking DNA and causing extensive damage.

In addition to oxidative damage, there are several hypothesized modifiable and non-modifiable risk factors for cancer including genetic predisposition, inflammation, obesity, insulin resistance, physical inactivity, and nutrition-related factors [7]. According to the previously published reports, about 75-80% of cancers are preventable by diet and lifestyle [41], and about 30% of cancer deaths may be attributed to diet alone [42]. Over the years, consumption of plant products, especially vegetables, have been postulated to be anti-carcinogenic [43]. Following sections will present an overview of the literature regarding the associations between vegetable intake and development of cancer. Because vegetables have many substances, which may have protective properties against cancer, potential mechanisms that may be underlying these associations will also be reviewed.

IV. Vegetable Consumption and Cancer: Evidence from the Literature

In 2007, the World Cancer Research Fund and the American Institute for Cancer Research (WCRF/AICR) released an extensive report of the evidence based on the publications from mid-1990s to 2007 investigating the associations of foods, nutrition, and cancer [7, 8, 44]. This report of the WCRF/AICR used certain classification terms to indicate the level of evidence regarding the associations of vegetable consumption and risk of cancer: "Convincing" represented the strongest level of evidence showing causal relationship, and "probable" represented the strong enough evidence to indicate probable causality. "Limited-suggestive" indicated presence of suggestive direction of the association but not strong enough to make a causal judgment.

The WCRF/AICR expert panel concluded that overall evidence about the protective role of vegetables against cancer risk was probable, but not convincing. In addition to the WCRF/AICR report, the International Agency for Research on Cancer (IARC) also evaluated the existing evidence about the associations of fruits and vegetables and risk for cancer [44]. Taken together, these expert reviews suggested that there was a likely protection resulting from higher vegetable consumption against certain site-specific cancers but not all types of cancers. For example, the review panel stated that the evidence for the protective role of non-starchy vegetable intake against the risk for cancers of the gastrointestinal tract, especially of mouth, pharynx, larynx, esophagus, and stomach, was probable. The evidence of inverse associations between the risks for nasopharyngeal, lung, colorectal, ovarian, and endometrial cancers and non-starchy vegetable intake was limited but suggestive. Similarly, there were other studies that suggested protective effects of carrots, allium vegetables, or other foods containing carotenoids, and vitamins C or E against some specific cancers [7].

Based on the evidence reviewed by the IARC [44], Vainio et al.[45], computed that approximately 5-12% of cancers could be prevented (preventable fraction) by a higher intake (e.g., highest quartile or tertile) of fruits and vegetables.

A summary of the results from the WCRF/AICR [7] and the IARC reports [44, 45] about the protective associations of vegetable consumption and various cancers is presented below and in Table 1.

Mouth and Pharynx:

This category includes the cancers of the mouth and all the associated organs, lips, tongue, cheeks, gums, palate, salivary gland, and vocal cords. Majority of the studies that investigated the associations between these cancers and non-starchy vegetables, raw vegetables, cruciferous vegetables, or leafy vegetables showed a decreased risk of cancer with increased intake of vegetables. Meta-analyses of four case-control studies suggested a 28% decreased likelihood of having cancer (OR: 0.72 95% CI: 0.63-0.82) with increments of 100g (~1 serving) increase in non-starchy vegetable consumption [7]. Similarly, meta-analyses of seven case-control studies by Vainio et al. noted almost 50% decreased likelihood of having oral and pharyngeal cancers (OR: 0.49; 95% CI:0.39-0.62) for high versus low vegetable intake [45].

Esophagus:

Majority of the studies showed a decreased risk of esophageal cancers with higher intake of non-starchy vegetables, although the associations were not always statistically significant. The meta-analysis performed by the WCRF/AICR [7] of the case-control studies showed a 13% decreased likelihood of having esophageal cancer with higher consumption of non-starchy vegetables (OR: 0.87; CI: 0.72-1.05), and a 31% less likelihood of having cancer with higher consumption of raw vegetables (OR: 0.69 95% CI: 0.58-0.83). The summary risk estimate computed by IARC showed a similar protective association (36% lower likelihood of having cancer) with higher vegetable intake in 12 case-control studies (OR: 0.64; 95% CI: 0.57-0.72) [45].

Stomach:

Changes in the stomach mucosal layers, due to both environmental factors and aging, may lead to atrophic gastritis, which may eventually develop into gastric cancer. Epidemiologic evidence, based on studies that evaluated total vegetables, green-yellow vegetables, green-leafy, or white vegetables, and non-starchy vegetables combined with fruits, generally showed decreased risk with increased vegetable consumption. Separate meta-analyses for non-starchy vegetables, green-yellow vegetables, white, and raw vegetables showed decreased risk levels ranging from 30% to 50% per 100g (~1 serving) increase in vegetable intake; the maximum decreased risk of 57% was detected per 100g (~1 serving) increase in the daily green leafy vegetable (lettuce and salad) consumption [7].

Additionally, it is noteworthy that there was a significant decreased risk in gastric cancer with increased consumption of allium-containing vegetables (onions, garlic, chives) [7]. Meta-analyses of case-control studies showed a 41% less likelihood of having stomach cancer for each additional serving of garlic per day (OR: 0.59; CI: 0.47 – 0.74) and about 23% less likelihood of having cancer for every 50g increase in total allium-containing vegetable consumption [7].

Conversely, a meta-analysis of six cohort studies by IARC showed no statistically significant association of stomach cancer risk and vegetable consumption; but a separate meta-analysis using 20 case-control studies indicated that there was a 44% less likelihood of having cancer (OR: 0.66 CI: 0.61-0.71) with higher vegetable intake [45]. There is no clear explanation for these differences in the results; however, recall bias in case-control studies could contribute to the differential finding.

Colorectum:

There is limited evidence suggestive of the potential protective role of vegetables, specifically non-starchy vegetables against colorectal cancer. According to the WCRF/AICR report, meta-analyses from 10 cohort studies showed no significant associations between the risk for colorectal cancers and non-starchy vegetable consumption; however, three of six case-control studies reported that higher garlic consumption significantly decreased risk of colon cancer (ranging from 10% to 79% decreased risk) [7]. Similarly, the IARC report of the meta-analyses using 18 case-control studies showed a 37% less likelihood of having cancer with high versus low vegetable intake (OR 0.63 95% CI: 0.56-0.70) [45].

Table 1: Summary of the evidence for vegetable consumption and cancer risk [7]

Cancer site	Non-starchy vegetables	Allium vegetables	Garlic
Larynx, Mouth, pharynx	🡻		
Nasopharynx	≈↓		
Esophagus	🡻		
Lung	≈↓		
Stomach	🡻	🡻	
Pancreas Gall bladder			
Liver			
Colorectum #	≈↓		🡻
Breast			
Ovary	≈↓		
Endometrium	≈↓		
Prostate			
Skin			

🡻: Indicates "probable" protective associations for the specified cancer sites for the type of vegetable.
≈↓: Indicates "limited suggestive" associations.
#: Indicates "probable" protective associations with intake of foods containing fiber.

Other cancers:

According to the WCRF/AICR report, there was a probable protective effect for lycopene-containing and selenium-containing foods and prostate cancer although these foods could also include non-vegetable sources of these compounds. The report indicated that there was limited evidence of protective associations between nasopharyngeal, lung, ovarian, and endometrial cancers and vegetable intake. The WCRF/AICR review did not find conclusive evidence for potential protective effects of vegetables and breast, gallbladder, kidney, bladder, or skin cancers. It is important to highlight that this extensive report also pointed out that there was no evidence to support detrimental associations for vegetables and risk for various cancers [7, 45].

V. Vegetable Consumption and Potential Protective Mechanisms Against Cancer

Vegetables are rich sources of antioxidant vitamins and minerals (e.g., beta-carotene, folate, and selenium), phytochemicals (e.g., indoles, isothiocynates, flavonoids, phenols, sterols, and allium compounds), and dietary fiber, which are hypothesized to be protective against cancer. Conversely, vegetables may also contain potentially harmful substances, which may contribute to the cancer risk. The potential mechanisms are presented in the sections below and summarized in Table 2.

Several vitamins in vegetables might be exerting protective effects against cancer. For example, carotenoids, which are precursors to vitamin A (retinol), are found in many vegetables but in higher concentrations in yellow, orange, and green leafy vegetables. The data from in vitro studies have shown that derivatives of vitamin A can reverse malignant changes [46]. Vitamin C, found in vegetables, such as broccoli, green peppers, cabbage, and tomatoes, has the potential to reduce nitrites in the stomach and scavenge free radicals, which are capable of causing oxidative damage [47]. In a cell-culture study, vitamin C (in conjunction with green tea extracts and two amino acids) has been shown to inhibit growth, invasion, metastasis, and angiogenesis of tumor cells [48]. Folate, found in broccoli, green leafy vegetables, and several types of beans, is another nutrient with antioxidant properties. Because folate also plays a role in DNA synthesis and cell replication [7], deficiency of folate may be related to increased chromosomal damage [49]. Vitamin E, found in green leafy vegetables and legumes, might have protective effects against cancer because it is a strong intracellular antioxidant [50], prevents damage to cell membranes, and it prevents the formation of N-nitroso-compounds, which are carcinogens [51].

Another group of dietary component that may be underlying the potential protective effects of vegetable intake against cancer is phytochemicals. Phytochemicals, including phenolics, carotenoids, and organosulphur compounds, are hypothesized to be anticarcinogenic by virtue of their antioxidative and antiproliferative properties, by influencing cell apoptosis and stimulating the immune system [36]. For example, phenolics, specifically flavonoids, have been linked to reducing cancer risk because of their antioxidative properties [52]. Among the vegetables commonly consumed in the US, phenolics are most commonly found in broccoli, spinach, onions, red peppers, carrots, cabbage, potatoes and celery [53]. Further, indoles, classified as organosulphur compounds, have been shown to modulate the effect of hormone-related cancers [43]. Indoles, phenols and coumarins found in vegetables are involved in stimulating the detoxification system [54]. However, evidence linking phytochemicals and cancer in human studies is not conclusive, probably because of the difficulties to accurately quantify these compounds in epidemiologic studies [55, 56].

Vegetables usually are a good source of fiber, and several mechanisms have been proposed for the potential protective role of fiber against cancer, specifically colorectal cancer. One of these mechanisms involves reduced transit time of fecal matter in the large intestine due to increased fecal bulk, which prevents carcinogens from being in the gut for long periods. Another proposed mechanism involves binding of fiber to carcinogens in the intestines and removing them from the colon [43]. Further, fermentation of fiber in the gut alters the pH and interferes with conversion of primary bile acids to secondary bile acids, which are adversely associated with cancer risk [43].

The potential protective effect of vegetables might also be linked to cancer through energy intake and obesity. Because vegetables usually have a low energy density, diets rich in vegetables may protect against obesity by providing a lower-energy diet overall. Additionally, diets with high amounts of vegetables may also be low in dietary fats. Diets high in meats, fatty foods and refined carbohydrates, which may attribute to higher body weight, are usually associated with lower levels of vegetable intake [7]. Overall, the literature suggests an adverse association between higher body weight and cancer risk and progression. For example, a recent large prospective study (n=46,349) reported that excess adiposity, specifically weight gain in adulthood, was associated with about 33% increased risk for colon cancer among men [57]. Several other studies, including a large, national population-based study (n=900,000) in the US, also support a higher risk of cancer mortality among overweight and obese individuals compared with those with normal body weight [58-60].

Despite these potential protective properties, vegetables might also have substances that might increase the risk of having cancer. For example, naturally occurring nitrates in vegetables are converted to nitrite in the body, and they may eventually form *N-nitroso* compounds that have tumor inducing properties specifically for cancers of the stomach or the gastrointestinal tract [43, 61, 62]. In addition to the naturally occurring components, certain food preparation methods can also introduce adverse effects: salt and salted foods have been linked to certain cancers (e.g., stomach cancer), and high consumption of salted or pickled vegetables may increase the risk for cancer [7, 63].

Table 2: Potential mechanisms of action between vegetable intake and cancer [7, 36, 43, 64]

Anti-carcinogenic mechanisms	*Pro-carcinogenic mechanisms*
Reduce antioxidant load	Nitrites
Scavenge free radicals	Salted or pickled vegetables
Decrease inflammatory response	
Reduce adiposity	
DNA repair	
Bind and remove carcinogens	
Stimulate the immune system	
Antiproliferation and differentiation	
Decrease chromosomal damage	
Detoxify carcinogens	
Inhibit carcinogen formation	
Provide low energy density	

In summary, current literature indicates the presence of several mechanisms that might be underlying the protective roles of vegetables against cancer. Although the latest expert reviews of the existing literature [7, 44] does not provide "convincing" evidence, these reports highlight several "probable" associations for the protective link between vegetable intake and various cancers.

There are several reasons that might have masked detecting the potentially existing associations. For example, the majority of the studies reviewed in these reports were case-control in design. It would be expected for individuals, who were already diagnosed with cancer, to change their diets and consume more vegetables, thereby attenuating the results of the study. Next, there are several other factors which are not captured by epidemiologic studies that may bias the results. For example, the nutrient content of vegetables would vary depending on the harvest, storage, packaging, the quantity of pesticides used, and soil, in which the vegetables were grown. Preparation and cooking methods may also influence the availability and absorption of food components. Lastly, it is possible that the adverse and protective effects of vegetables might negate each other. However, it is important to note that there was the body of epidemiologic evidence, which did not support detrimental associations of vegetable intake and risk for cancer.

Conclusion

This chapter presented an overview of the literature that examined the associations between vegetable intake, and type 2 diabetes and cancer. Currently, several studies point out the probable protective influence of higher vegetable intake against type 2 diabetes and various cancers. However, not all studies agree on this potential protective effect. Some of this disagreement might be coming from the methodological differences between the studies.

It is possible that various nutrients and non-nutrient components in vegetables and other foods might be exerting protective effects cumulatively. Additionally, diets high in vegetables might be replacing less healthful intake patterns or might be related to diabetes and cancer via complex relationships with other lifestyle characteristics and disease risk factors (e.g., obesity).

Regardless, the importance of vegetables in the diet should not be underestimated, especially considering that the expert reviews do not indicate any increased risk of type 2 diabetes or cancer in relationship to increased vegetable (i.e., non-starchy vegetable) intake. The WCRF/AICR expert panel recommends that the public health goals should be to consume approximately 600 g (~7 servings) of plant foods (includes both fruits and vegetables, specifically non-starchy vegetables) per day [7]. Similarly, the United States Department of Agriculture (USDA) recommends consumption of two cups of fruits and 2.5 cups of vegetables per day for a reference 2,000-calorie diet, and it emphasizes the importance of eating a wide variety of fruits and vegetables to obtain the most benefit from various nutrients [65]. The national estimates for 2003-2004 indicate that less than 50% of the US population consume three or more servings of vegetables per day [66]. Vegetable consumption, constituting less than 3% of total daily energy intake, is lower than the recommended levels globally as well [67]. Considering the high prevalence of type 2 diabetes and cancer, and the potential protective effects of vegetable consumption, aiming to achieve the vegetable intake levels that are recommended by the WCRF/AICR and USDA seems to be a valuable nutrition and public health strategy for most populations.

Acknowledgments

We would like to thank Maya Vadiveloo, MS, RD, Research Assistant at the Department of Nutrition, Food Studies and Public Health, New York University, for her support.

References

[1] CDC National Center for Health Statistics. Health, United States, 2007. [cited 2008 January 16]; Available from: http://www.ncbi.nlm.nih.gov/books/bv.fcgi?rid=healthus05.chapter.trend-tables

[2] Jemal A, Siegel R, Ward E, Hao Y, Xu J, Murray T, et al. Cancer statistics, 2008. *CA Cancer J Clin.* 2008 Mar-Apr;58(2):71-96.

[3] CDC. National diabetes fact sheet: general information and national estimates on diabetes in the United States, 2007. [cited Feb 3, 2009]; Available from: http://apps.nccd.cdc.gov/DDTSTRS/FactSheet.aspx

[4] World Health Organization. Diabetes. [cited February 3, 2009]; Available from: http://www.who.int/mediacentre/factsheets/fs312/en/

[5] Edwards BK, Howe HL, Ries LA, Thun MJ, Rosenberg HM, Yancik R, et al. Annual report to the nation on the status of cancer, 1973-1999, featuring implications of age and aging on U.S. cancer burden. *Cancer*. 2002 May 15;94(10):2766-92.

[6] Bennett P, Rewers M, Knowler W. Epidemiology of diabetes mellitus. In: Porte D, Sherwin, RS, ed. *Ellenberg & Rifkin's Diabetes Mellitus*. Stamford, CT: Appleton & Lange 1997:373-400.

[7] World Cancer Research Fund, American Institute for Cancer Research. Food, Nutrition, Physical Activity, and the Prevention of Cancer: A Global Perspective. Washington, DC: AICR 2007.

[8] American Diabetes Association. Diagnosis and classification of diabetes mellitus. *Diabetes Care*. 2008;31(Suppl 1):S55-S60.

[9] Anderson JW. Nutritional management of diabetes mellitus. In: Shils ME, Olson JA, Shike M, Ross CA, eds. *Modern Nutrition in Health and Disease*. 9th ed. Baltimore, MD: Lippincott Williams & Wilkins 1999:1365-94.

[10] Malecki MT. Genetics of type 2 diabetes mellitus. *Diabetes Res Clin Pract*. 2005 Jun;68 Suppl1:S10-21.

[11] Hu FB, Manson JE, Stampfer MJ, Colditz G, Liu S, Solomon CG, et al. Diet, lifestyle, and the risk of type 2 diabetes mellitus in women. *N Engl J Med*. 2001 Sep 13;345(11):790-7.

[12] Van Dam RM, Rimm EB, Willett WC, Stampfer MJ, Hu FB. Dietary patterns and risk for type 2 diabetes mellitus in U.S. men. *Ann Intern Med*. 2002 Feb 5;136(3):201-9.

[13] Ford ES, Mokdad AH. Fruit and vegetable consumption and diabetes mellitus incidence among U.S. adults. *Prev Med*. 2001 Jan;32(1):33-9.

[14] Montonen J, Knekt P, Harkanen T, Jarvinen R, Heliovaara M, Aromaa A, et al. Dietary patterns and the incidence of type 2 diabetes. *Am J Epidemiol*. 2005 Feb 1;161(3):219-27.

[15] Montonen J, Jarvinen R, Heliovaara M, Reunanen A, Aromaa A, Knekt P. Food consumption and the incidence of type II diabetes mellitus. *Eur J Clin Nutr*. 2005 Mar;59(3):441-8.

[16] Gittelsohn J, Wolever TM, Harris SB, Harris-Giraldo R, Hanley AJ, Zinman B. Specific patterns of food consumption and preparation are associated with diabetes and obesity in a Native Canadian community. *J Nutr*. 1998 Mar;128(3):541-7.

[17] Feskens EJ, Virtanen SM, Rasanen L, Tuomilehto J, Stengard J, Pekkanen J, et al. Dietary factors determining diabetes and impaired glucose tolerance. A 20-year follow-up of the Finnish and Dutch cohorts of the Seven Countries Study. *Diabetes Care*. 1995 Aug;18(8):1104-12.

[18] Villegas R, Shu XO, Gao YT, Yang G, Elasy T, Li H, et al. Vegetable but not fruit consumption reduces the risk of type 2 diabetes in Chinese women. *J Nutr*. 2008 Mar;138(3):574-80.

[19] Sargeant LA, Khaw KT, Bingham S, Day NE, Luben RN, Oakes S, et al. Fruit and vegetable intake and population glycosylated haemoglobin levels: the EPIC-Norfolk Study. *Eur J Clin Nutr*. 2001 May;55(5):342-8.

[20] Liu S, Serdula M, Janket SJ, Cook NR, Sesso HD, Willett WC, et al. A prospective study of fruit and vegetable intake and the risk of type 2 diabetes in women. *Diabetes Care*. 2004 Dec;27(12):2993-6.

[21] Williams DE, Wareham NJ, Cox BD, Byrne CD, Hales CN, Day NE. Frequent salad vegetable consumption is associated with a reduction in the risk of diabetes mellitus. *J Clin Epidemiol*. 1999 Apr;52(4):329-35.

[22] He K, Hu FB, Colditz GA, Manson JE, Willett WC, Liu S. Changes in intake of fruits and vegetables in relation to risk of obesity and weight gain among middle-aged women. *Int J Obes Relat Metab Disord.* 2004 Dec;28(12):1569-74.

[23] Hamer M, Chida Y. Intake of fruit, vegetables, and antioxidants and risk of type 2 diabetes: systematic review and meta-analysis. *J Hypertens.* 2007 Dec;25(12):2361-9.

[24] Dembinska-Kiec A, Mykkanen O, Kiec-Wilk B, Mykkanen H. Antioxidant phytochemicals against type 2 diabetes. *Br J Nutr.* 2008 May;99 E Suppl 1:ES109-17.

[25] Ford ES. Vitamin supplement use and diabetes mellitus incidence among adults in the United States. *Am J Epidemiol.* 2001 May 1;153(9):892-7.

[26] Liu S, Ajani U, Chae C, Hennekens C, Buring JE, Manson JE. Long-term beta-carotene supplementation and risk of type 2 diabetes mellitus: a randomized controlled trial. *Jama.* 1999 Sep 15;282(11):1073-5.

[27] Mayer-Davis EJ, Costacou T, King I, Zaccaro DJ, Bell RA. Plasma and dietary vitamin E in relation to incidence of type 2 diabetes: The Insulin Resistance and Atherosclerosis Study (IRAS). *Diabetes Care.* 2002 Dec;25(12):2172-7.

[28] Bazzano LA, Serdula M, Liu S. Prevention of type 2 diabetes by diet and lifestyle modification. *J Am Coll Nutr.* 2005 Oct;24(5):310-9.

[29] Larsson SC, Wolk A. Magnesium intake and risk of type 2 diabetes: a meta-analysis. *J Intern Med.* 2007 Aug;262(2):208-14.

[30] Ma B, Lawson AB, Liese AD, Bell RA, Mayer-Davis EJ. Dairy, magnesium, and calcium intake in relation to insulin sensitivity: approaches to modeling a dose-dependent association. *Am J Epidemiol.* 2006 Sep 1;164(5):449-58.

[31] Weickert MO, Pfeiffer AF. Metabolic effects of dietary fiber consumption and prevention of diabetes. *J Nutr.* 2008 Mar;138(3):439-42.

[32] Salmeron J, Manson J, Stampfer M, Colditz G, Wing A, Willett W. Dietary fiber, glycemic load, and risk of non-insulin-dependent diabetes mellitus in women. *JAMA.* 1997;277:472-7.

[33] Ludwig D, Pereira M, Kroenke C, Hilner J, Van Horn L, al. e. Dietary fiber, weight gain, and cardiovascular risk factors in young adults. *JAMA.* 1999;282(16):1539.

[34] Epstein LH, Gordy CC, Raynor HA, Beddome M, Kilanowski CK, Paluch R. Increasing fruit and vegetable intake and decreasing fat and sugar intake in families at risk for childhood obesity. *Obes Res.* 2001 Mar;9(3):171-8.

[35] Ledikwe JH, Blanck HM, Kettel Khan L, Serdula MK, Seymour JD, Tohill BC, et al. Dietary energy density is associated with energy intake and weight status in US adults. *Am J Clin Nutr.* 2006 Jun;83(6):1362-8.

[36] Liu RH. Potential synergy of phytochemicals in cancer prevention: mechanism of action. *J Nutr.* 2004 Dec;134(12 Suppl):3479S-85S.

[37] Ford ES, Will JC, Bowman BA, Narayan KM. Diabetes mellitus and serum carotenoids: findings from the Third National Health and Nutrition Examination Survey. *Am J Epidemiol.* 1999 Jan 15;149(2):168-76.

[38] Weinberg R. The biology of cancer. 1 ed. United States: Routledge 2006.

[39] Lopez-Lazaro M. Dual role of hydrogen peroxide in cancer: possible relevance to cancer chemoprevention and therapy. *Cancer Lett.* 2007 Jul 8;252(1):1-8.

[40] Khan N, Afaq F, Mukhtar H. Cancer chemoprevention through dietary antioxidants: progress and promise. *Antioxid Redox Signal.* 2008 Mar;10(3):475-510.

[41] Doll R, Peto R. The causes of cancer: quantitative estimates of avoidable risks of cancer in the United States today. *J Natl Cancer Inst.* 1981 Jun;66(6):1191-308.

[42] American Institute for Cancer Research / World Cancer Research Fund. Food, Nutrition, and the Prevention of Cancer: A Global Perspective. Washington DC: American Institute for Cancer Research 1997.

[43] Steinmetz KA, Potter JD. Vegetables, fruit, and cancer. II. Mechanisms. *Cancer Causes Control.* 1991 Nov;2(6):427-42.

[44] IARC. Fruit and Vegetables, IARC Handbook of Cancer Prevention. Lyon, France: IARC Press 2003.

[45] Vainio H, Weiderpass E. Fruit and vegetables in cancer prevention. *Nutr Cancer.* 2006;54(1):111-42.

[46] Prasad KN, Edwards-Prasad J. Expressions of some molecular cancer risk factors and their modification by vitamins. *J Am Coll Nutr.* 1990 Feb;9(1):28-34.

[47] National Research Council (US) Committee on Diet and Health. Diet and Health: Implications for Reducing Chronic Disease Risk: National Academy Press 1989.

[48] Roomi MW, Roomi N, Ivanov V, Kalinovsky T, Niedzwiecki A, Rath M. Inhibitory effect of a mixture containing ascorbic acid, lysine, proline and green tea extract on critical parameters in angiogenesis. *Oncol Rep.* 2005 Oct;14(4):807-15.

[49] MacGregor JT, Schlegel R, Wehr CM, Alperin P, Ames BN. Cytogenetic damage induced by folate deficiency in mice is enhanced by caffeine. *Proc Natl Acad Sci U S A.* 1990 Dec;87(24):9962-5.

[50] Kamal-Eldin A, Appelqvist LA. The chemistry and antioxidant properties of tocopherols and tocotrienols. *Lipids.* 1996 Jul;31(7):671-701.

[51] Lintas C, Lombardi-Boccia G, Nicoli S. Effect of cooking on availability and in vitro nitrosation of precursors of volatile N-nitroso compounds in seafood. *Food Addit Contam.* 1990 Jan-Feb;7(1):37-42.

[52] Russo GL. Ins and outs of dietary phytochemicals in cancer chemoprevention. *Biochem Pharmacol.* 2007 Aug 15;74(4):533-44.

[53] Chu YF, Sun J, Wu X, Liu RH. Antioxidant and antiproliferative activities of common vegetables. *J Agric Food Chem.* 2002 Nov 6;50(23):6910-6.

[54] Dragsted LO, Strube M, Larsen JC. Cancer-protective factors in fruits and vegetables: biochemical and biological background. *Pharmacol Toxicol.* 1993;72 Suppl 1:116-35.

[55] Ross JA, Kasum CM. Dietary flavonoids: bioavailability, metabolic effects, and safety. *Annu Rev Nutr.* 2002;22:19-34.

[56] Yang CS, Landau JM, Huang MT, Newmark HL. Inhibition of carcinogenesis by dietary polyphenolic compounds. *Annu Rev Nutr.* 2001;21:381-406.

[57] Thygesen LC, Gronbaek M, Johansen C, Fuchs CS, Willett WC, Giovannucci E. Prospective weight change and colon cancer risk in male US health professionals. *Int J Cancer.* 2008 Sep 1;123(5):1160-5.

[58] Calle EE, Rodriguez C, Walker-Thurmond K, Thun MJ. Overweight, obesity, and mortality from cancer in a prospectively studied cohort of U.S. adults. *N Engl J Med.* 2003 Apr 24;348(17):1625-38.

[59] Rodriguez C, Patel AV, Calle EE, Jacobs EJ, Chao A, Thun MJ. Body mass index, height, and prostate cancer mortality in two large cohorts of adult men in the United States. *Cancer Epidemiol Biomarkers Prev.* 2001 Apr;10(4):345-53.

[60] Siddiqui SA, Inman BA, Sengupta S, Slezak JM, Bergstralh EJ, Leibovich BC, et al. Obesity and survival after radical prostatectomy: A 10-year prospective cohort study. *Cancer*. 2006 Aug 1;107(3):521-9.

[61] Lin K, Wu Y, Shen W. Interaction of total N-nitroso compounds in environment and in vivo on risk of esophageal cancer in the coastal area, China. *Environ Int*. 2009 Feb;35(2):376-81.

[62] Takayama S, Thorgeirsson UP, Adamson RH. Chemical carcinogenesis studies in nonhuman primates. *Proc Jpn Acad Ser B Phys Biol Sci*. 2008;84(6):176-88.

[63] Kurosawa M, Kikuchi S, Xu J, Inaba Y. Highly salted food and mountain herbs elevate the risk for stomach cancer death in a rural area of Japan. *J Gastroenterol Hepatol*. 2006 Nov;21(11):1681-6.

[64] Steinmetz KA, Potter JD. Vegetables, fruit, and cancer. I. Epidemiology. *Cancer Causes Control*. 1991 Sep;2(5):325-57.

[65] United States Department of Agriculture. Dietary Guidelines for Americans. 2005.

[66] Sondik EJ. Healthy People 2010 progress review, focus area 19: nutrition and overweight. [cited February 3, 2009]; Available from: http://www.cdc.gov/nchs/about/otheract/hpdata2010/focusareas/fa19_2_ppt/fa19_2_ppt.htm

[67] Michels KB, Fuchs CS, Giovannucci E, Colditz GA, Hunter DJ, Stampfer MJ, et al. Fiber intake and incidence of colorectal cancer among 76,947 women and 47,279 men. *Cancer Epidemiol Biomarkers Prev*. 2005 Apr;14(4):842-9.

In: Fruit and Vegetable Consumption and Health
Editors: Anton Papareschi and Harvey Eppolito
ISBN: 978-1-60741-596-1

Chapter V

Elder Fruit Juices: Properties, Consumption, and Nutrition

J.E. Vlachojannis[1*], A. Schieber[2] and S. Chrubasik[3,4]
[1] Department of Orthodontics, Columbia University, New York, NY, USA
[2]Department of Agricultural, Food and Nutritional Science, University of Alberta, Edmonton, Alberta, Canada
[3]Institute of Forensic Medicine, University of Freiburg, Freiburg, Germany
[4]Herbal Medicines Research and Education Centre, Faculty of Pharmacy, University of Sydney, NSW, Australia

Abstract

A recent review of the literature has identified 19 *in-vitro* studies, 4 animal experiments and 3 clinical trials investigating elderberry fruit preparations. The effect profile of elderberry fruit covers antioxidative, antiviral, antiproliferative and possibly anti-inflammatory and antibacterial effects *in vitro*. One animal experiment indicated anti-inflammatory activity. One animal experiment and one clinical trial demonstrated a weak anti-lipidemic effect. The proprietary elderberry fruit product Sambucol[R] showed *in vitro* antiviral activity. However, the clinical evidence of antiviral effectiveness is presently only moderate because a confirmatory study is warranted. An increasing number of food supplements prepared from elderberry fruit go along with health claims. Consumers should therefore be fully informed about the benefits, risks and hazards associated with the consumption of elderberry fruit products.

The berries of European elder contain a number of health-promoting compounds. Since anthocyanins are absorbed in low quantities into the systemic circulation, they may

* Correspondence and requests for reprints to: Dr. Julia Vlachojannis, DMD, Columbia University, Department of Orthodontics, 630 W 168th, VC 9, Rm 219 B, NYC 10032, NY, USA, Tel. 0012123050698; FAX 0012123054609; email: jec2142@columbia.edu

be involved in beneficial effects. For transparency reasons, the anthocyanin contents should be declared on food supplements together with the method of analysis. HPLC with diode array and mass spectrometric detection appears to be the most reliable method for the determination of the profile and contents of anthocyanins present in such supplements, whereas spectrophotometric assays provide information only about the sum of compounds absorbing at a given wavelength. Using LC-MS, we showed that the anthocyanin content of a proprietary food supplement was negligible. Anthocyanins may be degraded during preparation of the food supplement by the impact of oxygen and heat or react with other constituents present. Selecting *Sambucus* genotypes rich in ascorbic acid and also in flavonols and anthocyanins - harvested at the optimum harvest time - may provide good quality raw materials to be processed into dietary supplements.

The daily doses of elderberry fruit or food products have not yet been systematically evaluated in dose-finding studies with respect to the specific effects. Berries may be toxic, especially for children, and also potentially allergenic. Anthocyanins may have an impact on urinary pH. Further studies are required to rule out that elderberry preparations interfere with renal stone formation. Preclinical safety data are urgently warranted.

Update on the Effect and Efficacy Profiles of Elderberry Fruit Preparations

The fruits of European elder (*Sambucus nigra* L., Fam. Caprifoliaceae) are used in traditional German medicine for their possible laxative, diuretic, diaphoretic and pain-relieving effects. Unfortunately, none of these effects has been investigated systematically. The fruits of European elder are therefore not monographed by the German Commission E (Blumenthal, 1998). A recent systematic review provides evidence that the above mentioned effects include antioxidative and antiviral activities and possibly anti-inflammatory, antibacterial and antiproliferative activities (Vlachojannis et al., 2009). The evidence is based on 19 *in-vitro* studies, 4 animal experiments and 3 clinical trials. Eleven studies investigated the radical-scavenging effect *in vitro* (Abuja et al., 1998; Pool-Zobel et al., 1999; Espin et al., 2000; Youdim et al., 2000; Roy et al., 2002; Lugasi et al., 2003; Wu et al., 2004; Ginsburg et al., 2004; Nakajima et al., 2004; Lichtenthäler et al., 2005; Cheng et al., 2007), and 4 studies dealt with the effect against various types of viruses such as influenza types A and B; n=1, Zakay-Rones et al., 1995), avian influenza; n=1 (Balasingam et al., 2006)), HIV; n=1 (Sahpira-Nahor et al., 1995), and herpes simplex-1; n=1 (Morag et al., 1997). Single studies investigated the antiproliferative (Thole et al., 2006), anti-inflammatory (Barak et al., 2002) and antibacterial (Chatterjee et al., 2004) effects, and another failed to demonstrate any muscle-relaxant effect of elderberry fruit extract in isolated porcine coronary arterial rings (Bell et al., 2006). The antiviral effect was also studied in chimpanzees (one exploratory study; Burge et al., 1999) and in humans (2 exploratory studies; Zakay-Rones et al., 1995; 2004). The randomized controlled studies in patients suffering from influenza were of good quality and provided moderate evidence of effectiveness. A confirmatory study is urgently needed to corroborate this result. Experiments in rats also showed that aqueous elderberry fruit extracts may decrease pentobarbitone-induced sleep induction time, may increase sleeping time and also enhance the effect of morphine, thus producing central depression and analgesia (Jacovljevic et al., 2000). An ethanolic extract may improve acetic acid-induced colitis (Bobeck et al., 2001). An elderberry concentrate with up to 3 mg anthocyanins/kg/day had little effect on cholesterol levels and fatty acid pattern in the liver of rats, but spared vitamin E (Frank et al., 2002). Only high doses of an elderberry concentrate (anthocyanidin consumption 4 g per day) showed some reduction in prostprandial serum lipids in humans (Murkovic et al., 2004).

In part based on these studies, in part because vegetable and fruit consumption is associated with less frequent Alzheimer morbidity (Dai et al., 2006), but also in part based on literature on the vasoprotective, neuroprotective and anti-aging effects of anthocyanins in general (Zafra-Stone et al., 2007; Kang et al., 2006; Galli et al., 2002), a number of food supplements advertise health claims for preparations from elderberry fruit. For example;

(a) Webpage: www.sambucol.com/index.cfm?id=506: Tested in clinical studies and trusted by millions worldwide, Sambucol® is the natural way to help your family stand up to winter's worst.
(b) Webpage: www.florahealth.com/flora/home/Canada/Products/8300.htm: Sambu elder concentrate provides the energy to feel great while the system rejuvenates. The Sambu Kit promotes detoxification through the liver, kidneys, colon and skin and in addition to the immune-supporting efficacy of elder, this plant helps to detoxify and revitalize the body. In this regard, elder has the following therapeutic properties: diuretic (elder flowers and berries greatly enhance the kidney activity, flushing out toxins and waste), expectorant (promotes the discharge of mucous and phlegm from the respiratory passages), diaphoretic (elder flowers and berries promote perspiration, which helps the body to release toxins), purifier (elderberries help purify the blood and kidneys). Sambucol was designed for anyone wanting to do a lengthened cleanse of the sinuses, skin, colon, lungs, kidneys and liver, it is used to release a toxic load from the body, it is helpful for anyone wanting to lose the excess weight of toxins and metabolic wastes, it is beneficial for mucous congestion, sluggish digestion or allergies and it is great for those unaccustomed to fasting but who still wish to cleanse.
(c) Webpage www.herbalremedies.com/elderberry.html: Elderberry juice concentrate is a non-alcoholic source for the health benefits of elderberries. A medically proven strong anti-viral and immune system enhancer, elderberry is recommended as part of a health maintenance program.

In view of the above mentioned studies and health claims, consumers should be fully informed about the benefits and risks and hazards associated with the consumption of elderberry fruit products.

The Active Principles in Elderberry Fruit

The active principle of the ripe berries of European elder has not yet been fully identified. However, a closer look at the co-active compounds takes away any doubts on the health-promoting effects of elderberry preparations. These compounds include: flavonols (e.g. hyperoside, isoquercitrin and rutoside; Figure 1), up to 1 % of anthocyanins, e.g. chrysanthemin (= cyanidin-3-*O*-glucoside), cyanidin-3-*O*,5-*O*-diglucoside, cyanidin-3-*O*-sambubioside, cyanidin-3-*O*-sambubioside-5-*O*-glucoside, sambucin (= cyanidin-3-*O*-rhamnoglucoside), sambucyanin (= cyanidin-3-*O*-xyloglucoside) (Figure 2), and traces of essential oil are among its co-active constituents. 100 g of fresh berries also contain vitamin B_2 (Figure 3; more than 60 mg), vitamin C and folic acid (Figure 3; about 20 mg), biotin and nicotinic acid amide (Figure 3; about 2 mg), and β-carotene, vitamin B_6 and pantothenic acid (Figure 3; less than 0.5 mg). However, unripe berries contain also toxic compounds, such as cyanogenic glycosides (e.g., sambunigrin (Figure 4), which is hydrolyzed in the gastrointestinal tract to release cyanide), and also lectines (Anonymous, 1994).

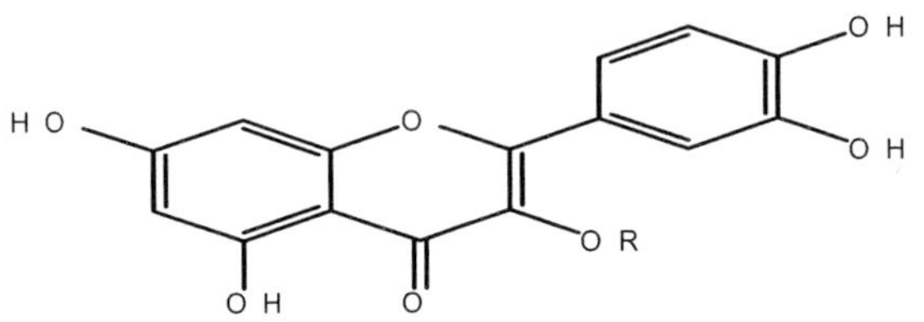

Hyperoside: R = Galactose
Isoquercitrin: R = Glucose
Rutin: R = Rutinose

Figure 1. Quercetin Glycosides

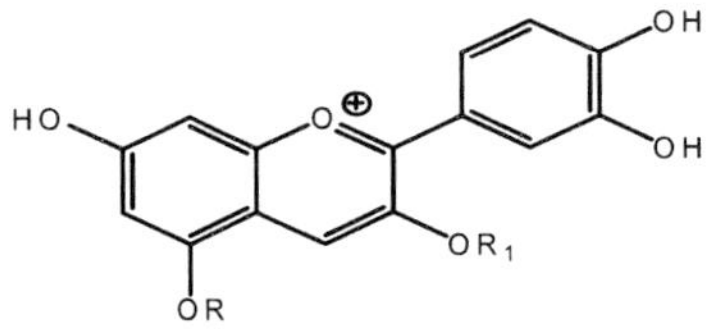

Chrysanthemin (Cyanidin-3-O-glucoside): R1 = Glucose, R = H
Sambucin (Cyanidin-3-O-rhamnoglucoside: R1 = Rhamnoglucose
Cyanidin-3,5-diglucoside: R, R1 = Glucose
Cyanidin-3-sambubioside: R1 = Sambubiose
Cyanidin-3-sambubioside-5-glucoside: R1 = Sambubiose, R = glucose
Cyanidin-3-rhamnoside: R1 = Rhamnose

Figure 2. Structure of cyanidin glycosides

Precondition for the effectiveness of elderberry fruit preparations

In order for anthocyanins to produce any clinical effect, they need to be absorbed from the gastrointestinal tract and reach the target cells. Youdim and co-workers (2000) demonstrated that elderberry anthocyanins are taken up into the membranes and cytosols of vascular endothelial cells, which subsequently effectively protected them against oxidative damage caused, for example, by hydrogen peroxide, dihydrochloreide or $FeSO_4$/ascorbic acid *in vitro*. After absorption from the gastrointestinal tract in mammals, anthocyanins were shown to be incorporated into plasma and liver in their intact glycoside forms (Miyazawa et al., 1999). Human pharmacological studies revealed very low gastrointestinal absorption of anthocyanidins after intake of a juice concentrate with 3.6 g or a berry extract with up to1852 mg anthocyanidins. Less than 1% of anthocyanidins were found in the urine (Bitsch et al., 2004; Frank et al., 2005, 2007). Within 4 hours after the intake of a berry extract containing up to 1600 mg anthocyanins, metabolites were detected in plasma and urine, along with small amounts of intact cyanidin-3,5-diglucoside (Cao et al., 1999, Milbury et al., 2002, Mülleder et al., 2002, Wu et al., 2002). Despite low absorption in humans, there is evidence that even low quantities of anthocyanins may modify markers of oxidative stress (Farombi et al., 2004).

Anthocyanidin content of elderberry food supplements

The nutritional benefit of elderberry fruits in the prevention of diseases depends on the net content of co-active compounds. Before any health claim is justified, the anthocyanin content needs to be determined and their stability assessed over time. The method of analysis needs explicitly be stated. For example, we investigated (i) a commercially available dietary supplement based on a juice concentrate which was prepared from 120 g of fresh berries and supplemented with flower juice and extract based on 3.9 g of dried flowers per 200 ml, consumed diluted in a ratio 1:5 (Chrubasik et al., 2008a), and (ii) a mother concentrate prepared in a ratio 6.5:1, maximum temperature used during processing was 90°C (Wild GmbH, Eppelheim, Germany). Anthocyanin contents were analysed by (i) the method described in the French Pharmacopoeia (Anonymous, 2000) using juice diluted in 0.1% MeOH-HCl at 528 nm; (ii) the pH-differential spectrophotometric method (absorption maximum of anthocyanins at 513 nm) described by Giusti and Wrolstad (www.does.org/masterli/facsample.htm) and, (iii) HPLC analysis with mass spectrometric identification of the cyanidin derivatives (Chandra et al., 2001; Kammerer et al., 2004).

Table 1. Anthocyanin contents of elderberry-based products as affected by the method of determination

Method	Dietary Supplement	Elderberry Juice Concentrate
French Pharmacopeia	762 mg/L	6400 mg/kg
pH Differential Method	85 mg/L	17200 mg/kg
HPLC-DAD	4 mg/L*	15400 mg/kg**

* cyanidin-3-glucoside (0.6 mg/L), cyanidin-3-sambubioside (2.2 mg/L) and cyanidin-3-sambubioside-5-glucoside (1.2 mg/L)

**cyanidin-3-sambubioside (13705 mg/kg), cyanidin-3-sambubioside-5-glucoside (1725 mg/kg); cyanidin-3-glucoside could not be quantified since it was superimposed by the predominant cyanidin-3-sambubioside peak, which might explain the slight difference of this result from the findings obtained from spectrophotometric determination of anthocyanins.

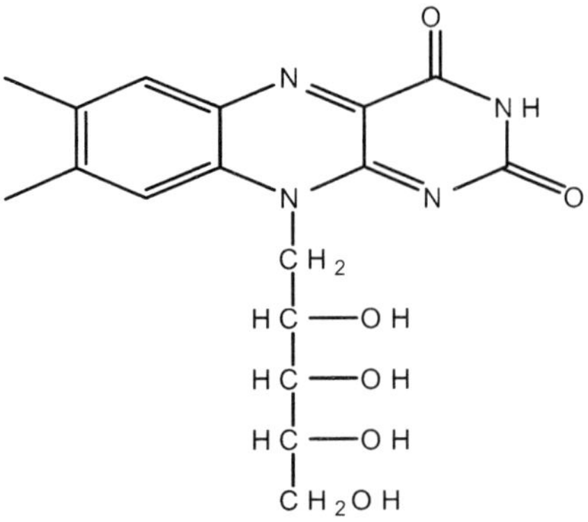

Vitamin B2

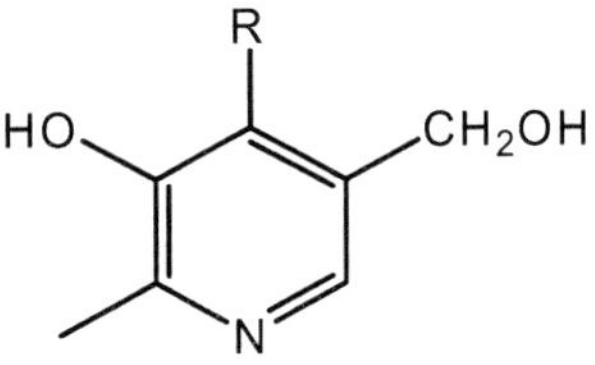

R=CH_2OH: Pyridoxine
R=CHO: Pyridoxal
R=CH_2NH_2: Pyridoxamine

Vitamin B6

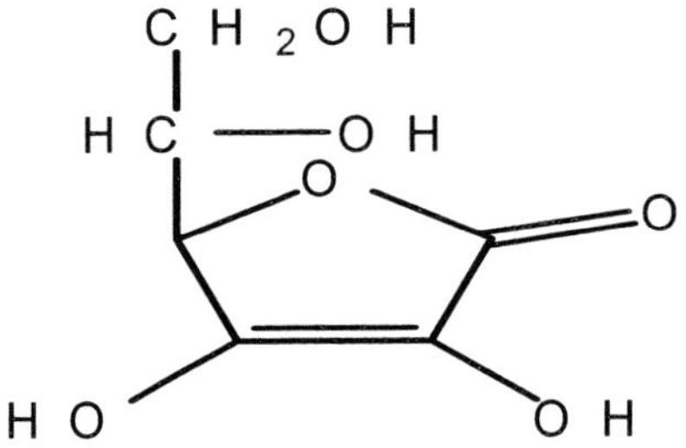

Vitamin C

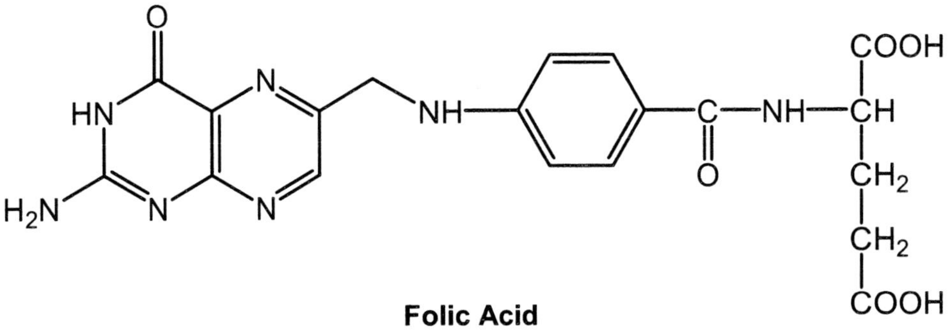

Folic Acid

Figure 3. (Continued next page)

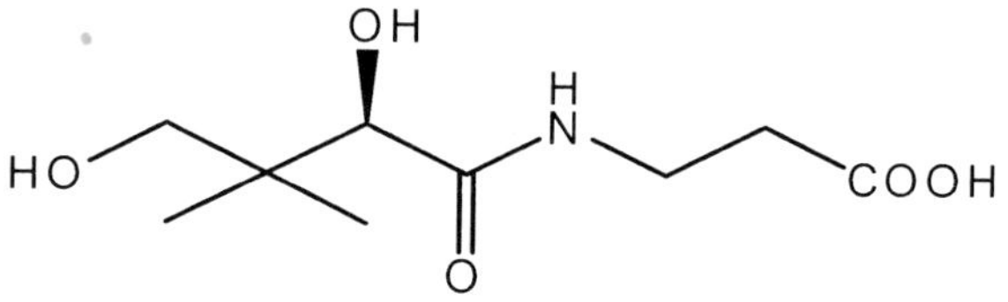

Pantothenic Acid

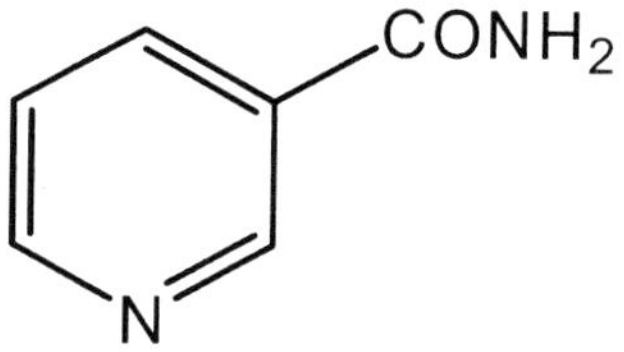

Nicotinamide

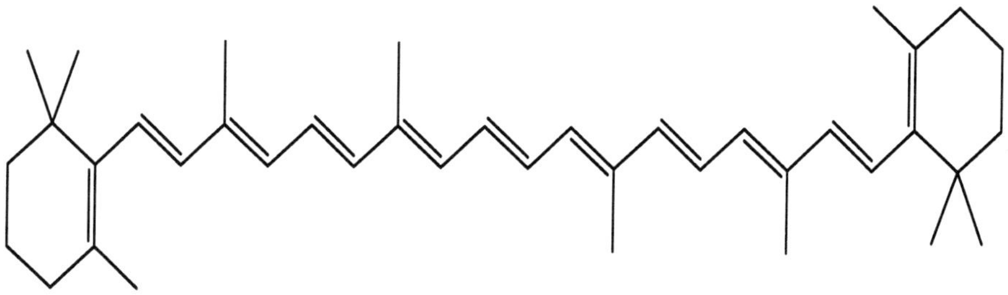

Beta-Carotene

Figure 3. Vitamine structures

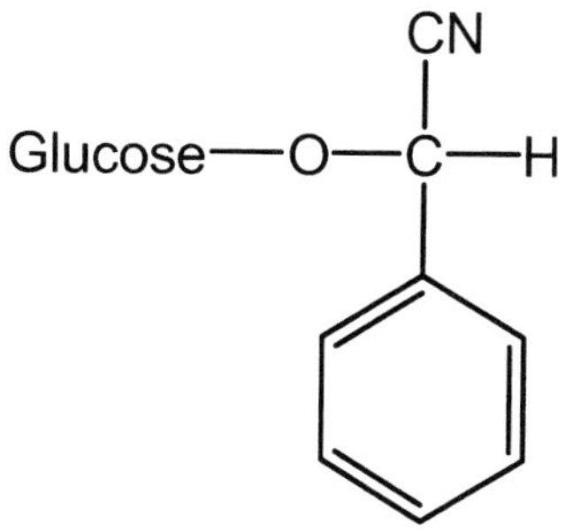

Sambunigrin

Figure 4. Structure of the toxic cyanogenic glycoside sambunigrin

The results are summarized in Table 1. The colour of the dietary supplement when diluted in water was reddish-brown with visual indication of oxidation (browning index 72%). The mother concentrate showed a bright red colour when diluted in water, with no visual indication of oxidation (browning index 24%). Table 1 indicates that the differing results obtained when different methods of determination were employed are more pronounced in the dietary supplement. Considering the high browning index of >70%, it is assumed that the sample was subjected to considerable thermal impact which finally led to the oxidation of phenolic compounds and the conversion of monomeric anthocyanins to coloured and non-coloured products. The French Pharmacopoeia method does not consider these conversions but measures all compounds absorbing at 528 nm irrespective of their chemical nature. In contrast, the pH differential method represents a fast and easy method for the quantitation of monomeric anthocyanins. Striking differences between the pH differential method and the HPLC method suggest that the samples have suffered from severe oxidative damage. During processing and storage anthocyanin contents may be reduced, either by degradation or by the formation of coloured derivatives, the so-called pyranoanthocyanins. Degradation may also be caused by oxidized phenolic compounds such as caffeic acid *o*-quinone. It remains to be established whether the chemically transformed anthocyanins possess any health-promoting or debilitating properties. Until this is proven, knowledge of the "true" anthocyanin content is mandatory to pre-estimate the potential antioxidative or antiaging effects of food supplements. Hyphenated techniques such as HPLC combined with diode array and mass spectrometric detection appear to be most reliable methods to detect active anthocyanins, especially if mother concentrates undergo further manufacturing processes (Chrubasik et al., 2008b). The health claims made for the proprietary elderberry concentrate (www.florahealth.com/flora/home/Canada/Products/8300.htm) cannot be related to its daily consumed anthocyanidin content and it remains to be established if the proclaimed health-promoting effects can be achieved with this food supplement.

Prerequisites for the Manufacture of Food Supplements with High Anthocyanin Contents

During processing, exposure to oxygen may destroy the anthocyanins (Kaack and Austedt, 1998). Likewise, heating (Sadilova et al., 2007) or storage at high temperatures (Heigl and Franz, 2003) result in degradation of the phenolic compounds and in decrease in the antioxidative capacity. Ascorbic acid may protect anthocyanidins but not quercetin from oxidative degradation (Kaack and Austed, 1998). Therefore, careful selection of appropriate raw material with a high content of ascorbic acid may be of advantage.

Enriching food supplements with phenolic compounds, in order to enhance health benefits, has been suggested (Vattem et al., 2005). However, it is still a matter of intense and controversial discussion whether such supplementation is clinically useful and as effective as concentrates of phenolics in their natural matrix. Selection of *Sambucus* genotypes may also help to obtain raw materials rich in health-promoting compounds.

Important quality characteristics such as content of phenolic acids and flavonoids are largely determined by the raw material (genotype), although other variables (ripening stage, process of juice production) do have some influence on juice yield and physicochemical characteristics like turbidity, titratable acidity, and soluble solids (Kaack et al., 2008). Factor analyses revealed correlations between the quality characteristics which may help manufacturers to identify the optimum *Sambucus nigra* genotype. Optimum time of harvest towards complete maturity was shown to be associated with maximum antioxidative capacity (Stefanovits-Banyai et al. 2004).

Daily Dosage

Elderberry juice or tea (aqueous extract): several cups per day.

For the preparation of tea, place 10 g dried berries into cold water for several minutes, then heat up slowly and boil shortly. Before filtering off, a drawing-time of 5 to 10 minutes is recommended (Anonymous, 1994).

Aqueous extract Sambucol^R: 4x2 spoons (15 ml) per day (Zakay-Rones et al., 1995; 2004).

All empirically recommended doses of food supplements including that of Sambucol^R have not yet been evaluated systematically. Dietary reference intake values do not exist for anthocyanins. A guideline on the optimal dose range for polyphenols is warranted which should be based on clinical studies demonstrating their health-promoting effects.

Adverse Events and Toxicity

The products investigated in the trials (Murkovic et al., 2004; Zakay-Rones et al., 1995; 2004) were well tolerated. Adverse events were not reported. However, consumption of a few ripe berries may cause emesis in children, and consumption of larger amounts of raw, insufficiently heated berries may produce nausea and emesis in adults (Anonymous, 1994; www.nlm.nih.gov/medlineplus/druginfo/herb_All.html#E), especially if the raw material accidentally contains unripe berries, leaves or bark. Reversible elderberry intoxication has been reported after several glasses of juice made from berries of *Sambucus mexicana.* The symptoms included nausea, vomiting, weakness, dizziness, and numbness. One person was hospitalized for stupor (www.cdc.gov/mmwr/preview/mmwrhtml/00000311.htm). Compounds responsible for the toxicity include cyanogenic glycosides (e.g. sambunigrin), which are hydrolyzed in the gastrointestinal tract to release cyanide, and also lectins (Anonymous, 1994).

In about 1% of 3668 patients tested, a skin prick test and/or radioallergosorbent test against ribosome-inactivating protein was positive (Förster-Waldl et al., 2003). The lectin type-2 ribosome-inactivating protein is the major elderberry fruit protein (Van Damme et al., 1997; De Benito et al., 1998, Gibres et al., 1996). Allergy to elderberry fruit products is, thus, possible, although not reported in the literature. Elderberry seed lectin is distinct from bark lectins (Peumans et al., 1991). Another lectin, *Sambucus nigra* agglutinin, was shown to induce the release of IL-4 from human basophils. As a result, IL-13 and histamine were released (Haas et al., 1999). Unfortunately, the toxic and allergenic lectins are of great importance for the elderberry antiviral (Chen et al., 2002; Vandenbussche et al., 2004) and potential antiproliferative (Citores et al., 2002) activities.

For elderberry preparations, preclinical safety data have not yet been carried out and are therefore urgently warranted, especially in light of the toxic lectins. Likewise, clinical safety data are needed for the elderberry food supplements in current use.

Does Elderberry Fruit Consumption Affect Renal Concrement Formation?

Some blackberry preparations may affect the urinary electrolyte composition and may interact with renal concretion formation. Consumption of a cranberry concentrate over 7 days, for example, has been shown to increase urinary oxalate, calcium, phosphate, and sodium (all lithogenic), but also urinary inhibitors of stone formation like magnesium and potassium (Terris et al., 2001). Supersaturation of uric acid was associated with a decrease in urinary pH (Kessler et al., 2002). In contrast, consumption of blackcurrant juice increased urinary pH and the excretion of citric and oxalic acids. The authors concluded that cranberry juice, due to its urine acidifying effect, might be useful in the treatment of brushite and struvite stones, whereas blackcurrant juice could support the treatment and metaphylaxis of uric acid stone disease because of its alkalizing effect. We recently showed that consumption of a proprietary elderberry fruit and flower concentrate had no impact on urinary pH and electrolyte consumption (Walz and Chrubasik, 2008). Due to the low quantity of anthocyanins found in the *Sambucus* concentrate (Chrubasik et al., 2008b), the study should be repeated with a *Sambucus* concentrate rich in anthocyanins before a final conclusion as to the impact of elderberry juice on urinary pH can be drawn.

References

Abuja PM, Murkovic M, Pfannhauser W. 1998. Antioxidant and prooxidant activities of elderberry (*Sambucus nigra*) extract in low-density lipoprotein oxidation. J Agric Food Chem **46**:4091-96.

Anonymous. 2000. French Pharmacopoeia 10th Edition. Monograph Folia *Vitis vinifera*.

Anonymous. 1994. *Sambucus nigra* L. In: Hagers Handbuch der Pharmazeutischen Praxis. Bd. 6, eds. Hänsel R, Keller K, Rimpler H, Schneider G. SpringerPress Berlin, Heidelberg, New York, pp 579-86.

Balasingam S, Lamkin R, Safirman D, Mumcuoglu M, Oxford JS. Neutralizing activity of SambucolR against avian NIBRG-14 (H%N1) influenza virus. 2006. IV. International Conference on Influenza, Preventing the Pandemic, Bird flu vaccines, London, June 23-24.

Barak V, Birkenfeld S, Halperin T, Kalickman I. 2002. The effect of herbal remedies on the production of human inflammatory and anti-inflammatory cytokines. Isr Med Assoc J **4** (11 Suppl):919-22.

Bell DR, Gochenaur K. 2006. Direct vasoactive and vasoprotective properties of anthocyanin-rich extracts. J Appl Physiol **100**:1164-70.

Bitsch I, Janssen M, Netzel M, Strass G, Frank T. 2004. Bioavailability of anthocyanidin-3-glycosides following consumption of elderberry extract and blackcurrant juice. Int J Clin Pharmacol Ther **42**:293-300.

Blumenthal M. 1998. The Complete German Commission E Monographs. The American Botanical Council, Austin, Texas.

Bobek P, Nosalova V, Cerna S. 2001. Influence of diet containing extract of black elder (*Sambucus nigra*) on colitis in rats. Biologia Bratislava **56**:643-648.

Burge B, Mumcuoglu M, Simmons T. 1999. The effect of Sambucol on flu-like symptoms in chimpanzees: prophylactic and symptom-dependent treatment. Int Zoo News **46**:16-19.

Cao G, Prior RL. 1999. Anthocyanins are detected in human plasma after oral administration of an elderberry extract. Clin Chem **45**:574-6.

Chandra A, Rana J, Li Y. 2001. Separation, identification, quantification, and method validation of anthocyanins in botanical supplement raw materials by HPLC and HPLC-MS. J Agric Food Chem **49**:3515-3521.

Chatterjee A, Yasmin T, Bagchi D, Stohs SJ. 2004. Inhibition of *Helicobacter pylori* in vitro by various berry extracts, with enhanced susceptibility to clarithromycin. Mol Cell Biochem **265**:19-26.

Chen Y, Peumans WJ, Van Damme EJ. 2002. The *Sambucus nigra* type-2 ribosome-inactivating protein SNA-I' exhibits in planta antiviral activity in transgenic tabacco **516**:27-30.

Cheng KW, Wu Q, Zheng ZP, Peng X, Simon JE, Chen F, Wang M. 2007. Inhibitory effect of fruit extracts on the formation of heterocyclic amines. J Agric Food Chem **55**:10359-65.

Chrubasik C, Maier T, Hofmann T, Torda T, Schieber A, Dawid C, Chrubasik S. 2008a. An observational study and quantification of the actives in a supplement with *Sambucus nigra* and *Asparagus officinalis* used for weight reduction. Phytother Res **22**:913-18.

Chrubasik S, Lüönd M, Schieber A. 2008b. Z Phythotherapie **29**:71-74.

Citores L, Ferreras JM, Muñoz R, Benítez J, Jiménez P, Girbés T. 2002. Targeting cancer cells with transferrin conjugates containing the non-toxic type 2 ribosome-inactivating proteins nigrin b or ebulin l. Cancer Lett **184**:29-35.

Dai Q, Borenstein AR, Wu Y, Jackson JC, Larson EB. 2006. Fruit and vegetable juices and Alzheimer's disease: the Kame Project. Am J Med **379**:464-475.

De Benito FM, Iglesias R, Ferreras JM, Citores L, Camafeita E, Méndez E, Girbés T. 1998. Constitutive and inducible type 1 ribosome-inactivating proteins (RIPs) in elderberry (*Sambucus nigra* L.). FEBS Lett **428**:75-9.

Espin JC, Soler-Rivas C, Wichers HJ, Garcia-Viguera C. 2000. Anthocyanin-based natural colorants: a new source of antiradical activity for foodstuff. J Agric Food Chem **48**:1588-92.

Farombi EO, Hansen M, Ravn-Haren G, Moller P, Dragsted LO. 2004. Commonly consumed and naturally occurring dietary substances affect biomarkers of oxidative stress and DNA damage in healthy rats. Food Chem Toxicol **42**:1315-22.

Förster-Waldl E, Marchetti M, Schöll I, Focke M, Radauer C, Kinaciyan T, Nentwich I, Jäger S, Schmid ER, Boltz-Nitulescu G, Scheiner O, Jensen-Jarolim E. 2003. Type I allergy to elderberry (*Sambucus nigra*) is elicited by a 33.2 kDa allergen with significant homology to ribosomal inactivating proteins. Clin Exp Allergy **33**:1703-10.

Frank J, Kamal-Eldin A, Lundh T, Maatta K, Torronen R, Vessby B. 2002. Effects of dietary anthocyanins on tocopherols and lipids in rats. J Agric Food Chem **50**:7226-30.

Frank T, Sonntag S, Strass G, Bitsch I, Bitsch R, Netzel M. 2005. Urinary pharmacokinetics of cyanidin glycosides in healthy young men following consumption of elderberry juice. Int J Clin Pharmacol Res **25**:47-56. **See** also: Bitsch R, Netzel M, Sonntag S, Strass G, Frank T, Bitsch I. 2004. Urinary Excretion of Cyanidin Glucosides and Glucuronides in Healthy Humans After Elderberry Juice Ingestion. J Biomed Biotechnol **2004**:343-345.

Frank T, Janssen M, Netzel G, Christian B, Bitsch I, Netzel M. 2007. Absorption and excretion of elderberry (*Sambucus nigra* L.) anthocyanins in healthy humans. Methods Find Exp Clin Pharmacol **29**:525-33.

Galli RL, Shukitt-Hale B, Youdim KA, Joseph JA. 2002. Fruit polyphenolics and brain aging: nutritional interventions targeting age-related neuronal and behavioral deficits. Ann N Y Acad Sci. **959**:128-32.

Giusti M, Wrolstad RE. 2000. Characterization and measurement of anthocyanins by UV-visible spectroscopy; www.does.org/masterli/facsample.htm.

Gibres T, Citores L, de Benito F, Inglesias R, Ferreras JM. 1996. A non-toxic two-chain ribosome-inactivating protein co-exists with a structure-related monomeric lectin (SNA III) in elder (*Sambucus nigra*) fruits. Biochem J **315**:343-344.

Ginsburg I, Sadovnic M, Oron M, Kohen R. 2004. Novel chemiluminescence-inducing cocktails, part II: measurement of the anti-oxidant capacity of vitamins, thiols, body fluids, alcoholic beverages and edible oils. Inflammopharmacology 12:305-20.

Haas H, Falcone FH, Schramm G, Haisch K, Gibbs BF, Klaucke J, Pöppelmann M, Becker WM, Gabius HJ, Schlaak M. 1999. Dietary lectins can induce in vitro release of IL-4 and IL-13 from human basophils. Eur J Immunol **29**:918-27.

Heigl D, Franz G. Stability testing on typical flavonoid containing herbal drugs. 2003. Pharmazie **58**:881-5.

Jakovljevic V, Popovic M, Mimica-Dukie N, Sabo J. 2001. Interaction of *Sambucus nigra* flower and berry decoctions with the actions of centrally acting drugs in rats. Pharmaceut Biol **39**:142-145.

Kaack K, Austed T. 1998. Interaction of vitamin C and flavonoids in elderberry (*Sambucus nigra* L.) during juice processing. Plant Foods Hum Nutr **52**:187-98.

Kaack K, Frette X, Christensen LP, Landbo AK, Meyer AS. 2008. Selection of elderberry (*Sambucus nigra* L.) genotypes best suited for the preparation of juice. Eur Food Res Technol **226**:843-55.

Kammerer D, Claus A, Carle R, Schieber A. 2004. Polyphenol screening of pomace from red and white grape varieties (*Vitis vinifera* L.) by HPLC-DAD-MS/MS. J Agric Food Chem **52**:4360-4367.

Kang TH, Hur JY, Kim HB, Ryu JH, Kim SY. 2006. Neuroprotective effects of the cyanidin-3-O-beta-d-glucopyranoside isolated from mulberry fruit against cerebral ischemia. Neurosci Lett **391**:122-6.

Kessler T, Jansen B, Hesse A. 2002. Effect of blackcurrant-, cranberry- and plum juice consumption on risk factors associated with kidney stone formation. Eur J Clin Nutr **56**:1020-3.

Lichtenthäler R, Marx F. 2005. Total oxidant scavenging capacities of common European fruit and vegetable juices. J Agr Food Chem **53**:103-110.

Lugasi A, Hóvári J. 2003. Antioxidant properties of commercial alcoholic and nonalcoholic beverages. Nahrung **47**:79-86.

Milbury PE, Cao G, Prior RL, Blumberg J. 2002. Bioavailability of elderberry anthocyanins. Mech Ageing Dev **123**:997-1006.

Miyazawa T, Nakagawa K, Kudo M, Muraishi K, Someya K. 1999. Direct intestinal absorption of red fruit anthocyanins, cyanidin-3-glucoside and cyanidin-3,5-diglucoside, into rats and humans. J Agric Food Chem **47**:1083-91.

Morag AM, Mumcuoglu M, Baybikov T, Schlesinger M, Zakay-Rones Z. 1997. Inhibition of sensitive and acyclovir-resistant HSF-1 strains by an elderberry extract in vitro. Phytoparasitica **25**:1.

Mülleder U, Murkovic M, Pfannhauser W. 2002. Urinary excretion of cyanidin glycosides. J Biochem Biophys Methods **53**:61-6.

Murkovic M, Abuja PM, Bergmann AR, Zirngast A, Adam U, Winklhofer-Roob BM, Toplak H. 2004. Effects of elderberry juice on fasting and postprandial serum lipids and low-density lipoprotein oxidation in healthy volunteers: a randomized, double-blind, placebo-controlled study. Eur J Clin Nutr **58**:244-9.

Nakajima JI, Tanaka I, Seo S, Yamazaki M, Saito K. 2004. LC/PDA/ESI-MS profiling and radical scavenging activity of anthocyanins in various berries. J Biomed Biotechnol **2004**:241-247.

Peumans WJ, Kellens JT, Allen AK, Van Damme EJ. 1991. Isolation and characterization of a seed lectin from elderberry (*Sambucus nigra* L.) and its relationship to the bark lectins. Carbohydr Res **213**:7-17

Pool-Zobel BL, Bub A, Schröder N, Rechkemmer G. 1999. Anthocyanins are potent antioxidants in model systems but do not reduce endogenous oxidative DNA damage in human colon cells. Eur J Nutr **38**:227-34.

Roy S, Khanna S, Alessio HM, Vider J, Bagchi D, Bagchi M, Sen CK. 2002. Anti-angiogenic property of edible berries. Free Radic Res **36**:1023-31.

Sadilova E, Carle R, Stintzing FC. 2007. Thermal degradation of anthocyanins and its impact on color and in vitro antioxidant capacity. Mol Nutr Food Res **51**:1461-71.

Sahpira-Nahor O, Zakay-Rones Z, Mamcuoglu M. 1995. The effects of Sambucol^{R} on HIV infection *in vitro*. Ann Israel Congress Microbiol, February 6-7.

Stefanovits-Banyai E, Schiffler E, Steger-Mate M, Sipos Bela Z, Hegedus A. 2004. A feketebodza (*Sambucus nigra* L.) beltartalmi értékeinek és antioxidáns hatásának változása az érés folyamán. 53. évfolyam **1**:33-36. www.mete.mtesz.hu/kiado/oszk/oszk_2004/2004-01/pdf/1_6.pdf

Terris MK, Issa MM, Tacker JR. 2001. Dietary supplementation with cranberry concentrate tablets may increase the risk of nephrolithiasis. Urology **57**:26-9.

Thole JM, Kraft TF, Sueiro LA, Kang YH, Gills JJ, Cuendet M, Pezzuto JM, Seigler DS, Lila MA. 2006. A comparative evaluation of the anticancer properties of European and American elderberry fruits. J Med Food **9**:498-504.

Van Damme EJ, Roy S, Barre A, Rougé P, Van Leuven F, Peumans WJ. 1997. The major elderberry (*Sambucus nigra*) fruit protein is a lectin derived from a truncated type 2 ribosome-inactivating protein. Plant J **12**:1251-60.

Vandenbussche F, Desmyter S, Ciani M, Proost P, Peumans WJ, Van Damme EJ. 2004. Analysis of the in planta antiviral activity of elderberry ribosome-inactivating proteins. Eur J Biochem **271**:1508-15.

Vattem DA, Ghaedianet R, Shetty K. 2005. Enhancing health benefits of berries through phenolic antioxidant enrichment: focus on cranberry. Asia Pac J Clin Nutr 14:120-30.

Vlachojannis JE, Cameron M, Chrubasik S. 2009. A systematic review on the *Sambucus* fructi effect and efficacy profiles. Phytother Res. 28:in press

Walz B, Chrubasik S. 2008. Impact of a proprietary concentrate of *Sambucus nigra* L. on urinary pH. Phytother Res 22:977-8.

Wu X, Gu L, Prior RL, McKay S. 2004. Characterization of anthocyanins and proanthocyanidins in some cultivars of *Ribes, Aronia*, and S*ambucus* and their antioxidant capacity. J Agric Food Chem **52**:7846-56.

Youdim KA, Martin A, Joseph JA. 2000. Incorporation of the elderberry anthocyanins by endothelial cells increases protection against oxidative stress. Free Radic Biol Med **29**:51-60.

Zakay-Rones Z, Varsano N, Zlotnik M, Manor O, Regev I, Schlesinger M, Mumcuoglu M. 1995. Inhibition of several strains of influenza virus in vitro and reduction of symptoms by an elderberry extract (*Sambucus nigra* L.) during an outbreak of influenza B Panama. J Alt Compl Med **1**:361-9.

Zakay-Rones Z, Thom E, Wollan T, Wadstein J. 2004. Randomized study of the efficacy and safety of oral elderberry extract in the treatment of influenza A and B virus infections. J Int Med Res **32**:132-40.

Zafra-Stone S, Yasmin T, Bagchi M, Chatterjee A, Vinson JA, Bagchi D. 2007. Berry anthocyanins as novel antioxidants in human health and disease prevention. Mol Nutr Food Res **51**:675-83.

In: Fruit and Vegetable Consumption and Health
Editors: Anton Papareschi and Harvey Eppolito
ISBN: 978-1-60741-596-1

Chapter VI

Loquat

Shunquan Lin
College of Horticulture, South China Agricultural University, China

Abstract

There are no FAO statistics available for loquat production and Consumption, thus, the present data derives from journal publication and from personal communications by experts in producing countries, especially from The 2nd Intern. Symp. on Loquat held at Guangzhou, China on April, 2006.

Loquat is now commercially produced in many countries. There are two big producing regions: eastern to southern Asia and around Mediterranean. The major producing countries are China, Spain, Pakistan, India, Japan and Turkey. China stands out as the main world producer of loquat with a crop area of more than 120,000 ha and annual production of 400,000 tonnes (t). Loquat are now grown in 20 out of 32 provinces, nearly all below 35°N.

The fruiting season now extends from December to Sep. due to incorporation of new regions. Loquat is frequently sold at local markets in China during the fruiting season, mainly from March to June, at a higher price. Fruits can be consumed fresh (more than 80%) or processed (about 5%) and can be used for jam, juice, wine, syrup, or as candied fruits; seeds are rich in starch (20 percent) and have been used to make wine. Loquat is highly nectariforous, with a heavy fragrance and high honey potential.

In Spain, as a consequence of environmental requirements, and for other socio-econnmic reasons, most of the production is located in three areas, namely, Alicante, Andalusia and Palancia. Loquat ripens between March and May, total production is 43,300 t, 36% of them is exported, which account for 85% of international trade of loquat. Loquats are concentrated in Japan's warm districts, including Kyushu and some prefectures of Honshu. Loquat is often the most expensive fruit on the market, reflecting the high cost of production, and is now marketed over a very long season. Although the crop area in Japan declined during and after World War II (only about 10 ,000t per year), protected culture has increased since the 1970s.

Leaves and fruits of loquats traditionally have been considered to have high medicinal value and there is evidence of pharmaceutically active compounds. An alcoholic extract has been shown to exhibit anti-inflammatory and hypoglycemic effects. Compared with some pomes sach as apple, pear and haw, and some tropical and subtropical fruits such as orange, banana, mango, litchi and longan, loquat fruits contained high levels of A vitamins, (537 μgRE), Carotene (322.3μg), Ca, Na and Se (20 Chemical composition of loquat fruit is presented in Table). A product contained loquat are recommended for chronhi bronchitis, coughs, and lung congestion. Contents are listed as loquat leaves with other herbs.

Besides common loquat (*Eriobotrya japonica* Lindl.), 20 other wild loquat species (such as *E. obovata, E. deflexa,*) in genus *Eriobotrya* are recently examined to have significant amounts of phenolics and flavonoids, and exhibit a strong antioxidant activity.

Introduction

Loquat (*Eriobotrya japonica* Lindl.), belonging to family Rosaceae subfamily Maloideae genus *Eriobotrya* which have more than 20 species, is a subtropical evergreen fruit tree that blooms in fall and early winter.

Records on loquat in China span over 2,000 years. The loquat cultivated in Japan was introduced from China in ancient times and loquat cultivation in Japan was described as early as 1180 (Ichinose 1995). People beyond eastern Asia first learned of the loquat from Kaempfer, who observed it in Japan and described it in *Amoenites Exotica* in 1712. In 1822, the English botanist, John Lindley, revised the genus *Mespilus*, and established loquat in a new genus, *Eriobotrya* (from Greek, *erio-*, wool, and *botrys*, a cluster, referring to the woolly, clustered panicles) (Huxley 1992). In 1784, the loquat was introduced from Guangdong into the National Garden at Paris, and in 1787 was introduced into the Royal Botanical Gardens at Kew, England. From this Beginning, loquat was distributed around the Mediterranean to various countries, including Algeria, Cyprus, Egypt, Greece, Israel. Italy, Spain, Tunisia and Turkey. Sometime between 1867 and 1870, loquat was introduced to Florida from Europe and to California from Japan. Chinese immigrants are assumed to have carried the loquat to Hawaii (Morton 1887). Cultivation spread to India and southeastern Asia, the East Indies, Australia, New Zealand, Madagascar, and South Africa. Loquats are now distributed in many Asian countries, for example, Laos, Nepal, Pakistan, South Korea, and Vietnam; in Armenia, Azerbaiian and Georgia; and in the Americas, including Argentina, Brazil, Chile, the mountains of Ecuador, Guatemala, Mexico, and Venezuela. Generally, loquats are found between latitudes 20 and 35° North or South, but can be cultivated up to latitude 45° under marine climates (Lin et al. 1999).

The specific epithet *japonica* was based on Thunberg's belief that the origin of loquat was Japan. In Chinese, loquat has two common names, *luju* and *biba* (southern Chinese) or *pipa* (northern Chinese). The Japanese name of loquat, *biwa*, is undoubtedly derived from the southern Chinese name, biba. Loquats cultivated in Japan were called Tang Biwa after the Tang Dynasty, 618--907. Common names of loquat in various languages in the world are often derived from the China name or loquat's former scientific name, mispilus, or medlar. The English name, loquat, is derived from the Chinese luju, while the present names in French are *bibassier*, derived from *biba*, or *nefiier du Japon*, literally medlar of Japan. The names in Spanish, German, and Italian are all derived from *mespilus* e.g., *nispero japones*, *japanische mispel*, and *nespola giapponese*, respectively (Morton 1987). In Portugal, loquat is called *ameixa do Japao*, or plum of Japan.

Table 1. Loquat species and their varieties and forms.

	Eriobotrya species	Representative area
1	*E.angustissima* Hook. f	Laos, Southern Vietnam
2	*E. bengalensis* Hook.f.	South-western China
3	f. *angustifolia* Vidal	Yunnan, China
4	f. *contract* Vidal	Vietnam; Yunnan,China
5	f. *intermedia* Vidal	Yunnan, China
6	*E. cavaleriei* Rehd	Guangdong, China
7	*E. deflexa* Nakai	Taiwan,China
8	var. *buisanensis* Nakai	Taiwan,China
9	var. *koshunensis* Nakai	Taiwan,China
10	*E. elliptica* Lindl.	Tibet, China
11	var. *petelottii* Vidal	Vietnam
12	f. *petiolata*	Tibet, China
13	*E. fragrans* Champ	Guangdong, China
14	var. *furfuracea.* Vidal	Vietnam
15	*E. henryi* Nakai	Yunnan, China
16	*E. hookeriana* Decne	Tibet, China
17	*E. japonica* Lindl.	Asia and around Mediterranean
18	*E .kwangsiensis* Chun	Guangxi,China
19	*E.latifolia* Hook.	Moalmayne
20	*E.macrocarpa* Kurz	Burma
21	*E. malipoensis* Kuan	Yunnan, China
22	*E. obovata* W.W.Smith	Yunnan, China
23	*E. philippinensis* Vidal	Philippines
24	*E. poilanei* Vidal	Vietnam
25	*E. prinoides* Rehd and Wils	Yunnan, China
26	var. *laotica* Vidal	Laos
27	var. *dadunensis* H.Z.Zhang	Sichuan China
28	*E. salwinensis* Hand-Mazz	Yunnan, China
29	*E. seguinii* Card	Guangxi,China
30	*E. serrate* Vidal	Yunnan, China
31	*E.stipularis* Craib	Cambodge
32	*E. tengyuehensis* W.W.Smith	Yunnan, China

Eriobotrya is often confused with *Mespillus*, and sometimes with *Crataegus* and *Photinia*. So, the number of loquat species had been under dispute and the opinions of authors in different countries vary. Now, we know that there are at least 22 species and 10 their varieties or forma. Most of them originated in southern China, the rest originated in Southeastern Asia (Table 1). Among them, only is *E. japonica* Lindl widely used as a cultivated fruit tree, though some of them can be used as stock, others used as Chinese medicine.

The main characteristics of the genus *Eriobotrya* are as follows (Huxley 1992): leaves alternate, simple, coriaceous, coarsely dentate; petiole short; flowers small, white, in broad pyramidal, usually densely lanate-pubescent, terminal panicles; bracts deltoid-ovate, persistent; calyx 5-lobed, acute, persistent; petals 5, ovate to suborhicular, clawed; stamens 20-40; styles 2-5, basally connate; ovary inferior, each locule 2-ovulate. Fruit an ohovoid to globular pome, with persistent calyx lobes at apex; seeds (1-9) are large.

Yu (1979) described the main characteristics of *E. japonica* as follows: evergreen tree, occasionally up to 10 m; shoot density varies with cultivar. Leaves on upper surface usually lustrous, lower surface often with pubescence; blades are narrow or broad, 12-30 cm long and 3-9 cm wide. Inflorescence 10-19 cm long, the main panicle axis bears 5-10 branched secondary axes, with 70-100 flowers, occasionally more than 100; hermaphrodite, flower size 12-20 mm. Fruit shape in longitudinal section as round, obovate, or elliptical; fruit size 2-5 cm; average weight usually about 30-40 g. same cultivars such as 'Jiefangzhong' average 70 g, the largest one 172 g, Spainish cultivar ‘Marc’ average 90 g, the largest one weigher than 200 g. peal and flesh white or yellow; fruit apex concave, flat or convex, with calyx cavity closed or open; ease of fruit peeling depending on cultivars; thickness of flesh 0.5-0.8 cm, proportion of flesh usually 60-80%; Brix value 6.5-17°, some cultivars such as 'Huangyang No. 5' higher than 20°; number of seeds 1-8, often 3-4, each seed weight 1.1-3.6 g. The loquat has relatively large seeds, as the subfamily Amygdaloideae, but has multiple seeds as do the subfamiles Rosoideae and Maloideae.

Loquat Consumption

Consumption lies on production.

There are no FAO statistics available for loquat production, thus the present data derives from journal publication and from personal communications by experts in producing countries, and mostly from The 2nd International Symposium on Loquat held at Guangzhou, China on April, 2006. We further collect the statistics (Table 2) which includes countries where the crop area of loquat exceeds 30 ha. China stands out as the main world producer of loquat with a crop area of more than 118,000 ha and annual production of 454,000 tonnes (t). Loquat are now grown in 20 out of 32 provinces, nearly all below 35°N. Production of loquat in the main provinces in China is also presented in Table 2. Sichuan is the leading producing province.

Spain is the second loquat producer in the world after China. However, Spain accounts for 84% of international trade, the international trade in loquat is very low (about 8% of total production). Although some growers market their own production, most growers are

Table 2. The area and production of loquat in main countries (left) and in main provinces of China (right). Countries are included where cultivated area exceeds 30 ha.

Main countries				China			
Country	Area (1000 ha)	Production (1000 t)	Notes	Province	Area (1000 ha)	Production (1000 t)	Leading cultivar
China	118.27	453.6		Sichuan	50	210.0	Dawuxing, Longquan No. 1
Spain	3.023	43.30	Export	Fujian	25.1	94.9	Zaozhong No. 6, Jiefangzhong
India	3			Chongqing	13.2	20.5	Dawuxing
Japan	2.05	9.24		Zhejiang	9.6	64	Dahongpao, Luoyangqing, Ruantiaobaisha
Pakistan	1.38	9.87		Hunan	5.3	16	Dawuxing, Dahongpao
Turkey	0.82	12.00	Export	Guangdong	3.3	18	Zaozhong No. 6, Chonghong No. 3
Italy	0.66	4.41		Guizhou	3	3.5	Dahongpao, Luoyangqing
Morocco	0.38	6.40		Jiangxi	2	10	Zhuluobaisha, Zhuluohongsha
Israel	0.33	3.00		Shanxi	2	0.6	Jiefangzhong, Dawuxing
Greece	0.3	2.75		Guangxi	1.2	3.2	Banhong, Dawuxing
Brazil	0.3	2.40		Taiwan	1		Tanaka, Mogi
Portugal	0.24	0.95		Anhui	0.8	6	Dahongpao, Guangrong, Caobao
Chile	0.14	0.30	Export	Jiangsu	0.7	5.4	Baiyu, Qingzhong, Guanyu
				Shanghai	0.67	0.5	Baiyu, Guanyu
				Hubei	0.3	1	
				Gansu	0.1		
Total	130.89	548.22			118.27	453.6	

Table 3. Harvest season of loquat in China

Location	Cultivar	Jan.	Feb.	March	April	May	June	July	Aug.	Sep.	Oct.	Nov.	Dec.
Panxi, Sichuan Mengzi,Yunnan	Zaozhong No.6	——											
Panxi, Sichuan	Zaozhong No.6		——										
Guangdong Fujian	Zaozhong No.6			——									
Guangdong Fujian	Zaozhong No.6				——								
Fujian zhejiang Chengdu,Sichuan Jiangsu	Jiefangzhong Ruantiaobaisha Dawuxin Baisha					——							
Chengdu,Sichuan Jiangsu	Dawuxin Baisha						——						
Aba, Sichuan	Dawuxin							——					
Aba, Sichuan	Dawuxin								——				
Aba, Sichuan	Dawuxin									——			
Panxi, Sichuan	Zaozhong No.6												——

organized in association. In these associations, individual growers bring their production classified and packed. Spain exports 36-47% of total production. While production is exported to many countries, more than 80% of the export is destined for Italy, Portugal and France.

Although China stands out as the first world producer of loquat, Spain is the biggest consumption per capita as well as export. The crucial factor is population. China has about 1300 million people, Spain has about 40 million. The Chinese consumed 0.3 Kg per capita per year, while Spanish consumed 0.6 Kg per capita per year though Spain exported about 40% of production to other countries.

Besides Spain, Turkey and Chile exported 10% to 20% of total production 12,000 t to some countries such as Saudi Arabia, Kuwait, Jordan, Russia, Sweden and Germany. Chile exported some of loquat (their total production is 300 t) to the United States. China exported a small quantity of production (1% - 5%, unstable) to Hongkong and Singapore.

The fruiting season in China now extends from December to Sep. due to incorporation of new regions. The harvest season in various regions by various cultivar are shown in Table 3. However, more than 50% of China loquat mature in May in Fujian, Sichuan and Zhejiang. Loquat is frequently sold at local markets in China during the fruiting season, at a higher price, About 10 Yuan (about 1.5 $) per Kg, higher than a lot of fruits in normal harvest seasons such as peach in May, Litchi in June and July, Longan in July and August, Banan, Citrus, Orange, Mango, Apple, Pear, Grape in anytime. Price of loquat generally is similar to that of bayberry (*Myricaceae rubra* Sieb. Et Zucc.), Chinese white olive [*Canarium album* (Lour.) Raeusch] and Java rose-apple [*Syzygium samarangensis* (Bl.) Merr. Et Perry].

Most of loquats (more than 80%) in China be consumed by fresh fruits. Because of quite higher price of fresh fruit, few loquat be stored by CA or other storage method (Yonghua, Z, et al., 1993). The fruit matured in later season in Jiangsu and Sichuan sometime are stored by CA for month, few people like them, too expensive, and taste is not very good. Besides fresh fruit, loquat can be consumed by a lot of forms, by processed (lower than 5%) and can be used for jam, juice, wine, syrup, or as candied fruits; seeds are rich in starch (20 percent) and have been used to make wine. There are no statistics available for canned industry in China, in leading producing area Fujian and Sichuan, farmer often make some cans by themselves for their family and their relatives. During 70's and 80's in last century, loquat fresh fruit is so cheap that about 20% to 30% of loquat fruits have been used as loquat cans, from 90's to now the price of loquat is higher and higher, the canned industry is smaller and smaller.

In Spain, loquat processing also produces juice, liquor, fruit canned in syrup and jam. The amount of fruit used for industry depends on the crop year. Only those fruits unsuitable for fresh market are used by the industry with the amount ranging between 10 to 20% of total production. The canned industry produces an average of 100 tons per year (Caballero and Fernández, 2004).

Loquat for Human Health

Chemical composition of loquat fruit is presented in Table 4(Church et al. 1935) . In various cultivars, sucrose, sorbitol, glucose, and fructose varied almost 6-fold, but total sugars varied less than 2-fold (Hirai 1980; Uchino et al. 1994b). Loquat flesh contained 0.42 g crude protein/100g fresh wt, 146 mg essential and 387 mg total amino acids. Ten essential amino acids were measured, with leucina the most abundant and cysteine-cystine the least abundant. Of the eight nonessential amino acids measured, glutamic and aspartic acids were the most abundant, with an unusually high level of proline (9.7 g per 100 g recovered amino acids). The carotanoids of loquat fruit are mainly responsible for flesh and skin color, which varied from yellowish white, yellow to deep orange (Godoy and Amaya 1995). Total carotenoid values, especially carotene, vary widely in flesh fruit peel and pulp. Total carotenoid values in the peel are several times higher than in the pulp. The content of carotene in yellow-orange fruit was 0-10 times higher than in the yellow-white fruits, while the contents of zeaxanthin, hitein, and violaxanthln in yellow-orange fruit were much lower. Eighteen volatile compounds were identified in a methylene chloride extract of a distilled fraction from loquat fruit. The major components are phenylethyl alcohol, 3-hydroxy-2-butanone, phenylacetadehyde, and hexen-1-ols.

Table 4. Chemical composition of loquat (Church et al. 1935).

Variable	Champagne	Advice	Thales
Moisture (%)	85.0	84.7	86.1
Total solids (%)	15.0	14.3	13.9
Insoluble solids (%)	2.3	2.7	2.4
Soluble solids (%)	12.7	11.6	11.5
Total acid (%)	0.4	0.5	0.7
Total malic acid (%)	0.3	0.3	0.5
Protein (%)	0.4	0.4	0.4
Ether extract (%)	0.2	0.2	0.2
Reducing sugars (%)	6.7	5.7	6.1
Sucrose (%)	3.4	3.4	2.4
Total sugar (%)	10.1	9.1	8.5
Alcohol ppt (%)	0.6	0.7	0.9
Pectic acid (%)	0.3	0.4	0.4
Total ash (%)	0.5	0.5	0.5
Soluble ash (%)	0.4	0.4	0.4
Insoluble ash (%)	0.1	0.1	0.1

Fruit composition of loquat compared with those of some pome fruits and tropical and subtropical fruits (Yuexin Y 2004) are shown in Table 5. From the table, we can know that Compared with some pomes such as apple, pear and haw, and some tropical and subtropical fruits such as orange, banana, mango, litchi and longan, loquat fruits contained high levels of A vitamins, (537 μgRE), Carotene (322.3μg), Ca, Na and Se.

Table 5. Fruit composition of loquat compared with those of some pome fruits and tropical and subtropical fruits (Yuexin Y 2004)

Fruit	Energy (kcal)	Protein (g)	Fat (g)	CHO (g)	Dietary Fiber(g)	VitA (μgRE)	Carotene (μg)	Vit B_1 (mg)	Vit B_2 (mg)	Vit C (mg)	Vit E (mg)	Ca (mg)	P (mg)	K (mg)	Na (mg)	Mg (mg)	Fe (mg)	Zn (mg)	Se (μg)
Apple	52	0.2	0.2	13.5	1.2	3	20	0.06	0.02	4	2.12	4	12	119	1.6	4	0.6	0.19	0.12
Pear	44	0.4	0.2	13.3	3.1	6	33	0.03	0.06	6	1.34	9	14	92	2.1	8	0.5	0.46	1.14
Haw	95	0.5	0.6	25.1	3.1	17	100	0.02	0.02	53	7.32	52	24	299	5.4	19	0.9	0.28	1.22
Loquat	39	0.8	0.2	9.3	0.8	537	3223	0.01	0.03	8	0.24	17	8	122	4.0	10	1.1	0.21	0.72
Orange	47	0.8	0.2	11.1	0.6	27	160	0.05	0.04	33	0.56	20	22	159	1.2	14	0.4	0.14	0.31
Banana	91	1.4	0.2	22.0	1.2	10	60	0.02	0.04	8	0.24	6	18	330	1.3	29	0.3	0.16	0.81
Mango	32	0.6	0.2	8.3	1.3	150	897	0.01	0.04	23	1.21	Tr	11	138	2.8	14	0.2	0.09	1.44
Litchi	70	0.9	0.2	16.6	0.5	2	10	0.10	0.04	41	-	2	24	151	1.7	12	0.4	0.17	0.14
Longan	71	1.2	0.1	16.6	0.4	3	20	0.01	0.14	43	-	9	30	248	3.9	10	0.2	0.40	0.83

Loquat is highly nectariforous, with a heavy fragrance and high honey potential. Loquat blooms in late autumn and early winter, few fruit tree even plant bloom in this season the Northern Hemisphere, it is cold and dry, it is believed that the quality of loquat honey is supreme good so that the honey is sold very expensively.

Leaves and fruits of loquats traditionally have been considered to have high medicinal value (Duke and Ayensu 1985; Wee and Hsuan 1992) and there is evidence of pharmaceutically active compounds (Morton 1987; Noreen et al. 1988; Chen et al. 1991; DeTommasi 1992). The ether-soluble fraction of the ethanolic extract of the leaves showed anti-inflammatory activity when applied topically to rats (Sinmizu et al. 1986). An alcoholic extract has been shown to exhibit anti-inflammatory and hypoglycemic effects. Loquat fruits contained low levels of B vitamins, including thimine, riboflavin, and niacin (Shaw and Wilson 1981). For at least 50 years, Chinese food stores in the United States have sold a product imported from Hong Kong and recommended for chronhi bronchitis, coughs, and lung congestion. Contents are listed as loquat leaves with other herbs (Duke and Ayensu 1985; Wee and Hsuan 1992).

Besides common loquat (*Eriobotrya japonica* Lindl.), other wild loquat species (such as *E. obovata*, *E. deflexa*,) in genus *Eriobotrya* are recently examined to have significant amounts of phenolics and flavonoids, and exhibit a strong antioxidant activity. The difference in contents of phenolics and flavonoids could be due to the different genotypes. It is expected that the wild germplasm can be utilized better as an important source of pharmacological agents by evaluating their antioxidant activities (Yanping H, et al., 2007). Of the 12 *Eriobotrya* species examined in their study, *E. obovata* exhibited the highest content of total phenolics and flavonoids, and the strongest antioxidant activity in the leaf tissues, followed by *E. deflexa*, *E. prinoides*, *E. deflexa* var. koshunensis, *E. elliptica* and *E. bengalensis*. Furthermore, the significant correlation existed between the content of total phenolics or flavonoids and free radical scavenging activity or reducing power. The study suggests that some wild species being higher in contents of total phenolic and flavonoids as well as stronger antioxidant activity might have a potential utilization value.

Conclusion

There are two big regions for commercial loquat production: eastern to southern Asia and around Mediterranean. The major producing countries are China and Spain, respectively. China stands out as the main world producer of loquat with annual production of 454,000 tonnes (t), Spain have annual production of 43,300 t. Total of both is 496,000 t and accounts for more than 90% of world total production (549,220 t). However, loquat is frequently sold at local markets in China during the fruiting season and consumed fresh (more than 80%) or processed (about 5%) and can be used for jam, juice, wine, syrup, or as candied fruits; while in Spain, 36% of total production is exported to Italy, Portugal or France. Because of cultivating loquat spend much more labors (flower-thinning, fruit-thinning, bag-covering and fruit-picking and so on, cost of labor is 2/3 of total cost) , fresh loquat fruit is quite expensive, few loquat fruit be stored by CA or other storage method or processed, for the product is more expensive, therefore, loquats are mainly consumed by fresh, loquat production mainly increase in developing country where labor is relatively cheaper.

Loquat fruits are not only tasty but also nutritious and healthy. And, leaves of loquats traditionally have been considered to have higher medicinal value, but for tasty, leaf and fruit are often mixed for Chinese medicine, and there is evidence of pharmaceutically active compounds. Besides common loquat (*Eriobotrya japonica* Lindl.), 20 other wild loquat species (such as *E. obovata, E. deflexa,*) in genus *Eriobotrya* are recently examined to have significant amounts of phenolics and flavonoids, and exhibit a strong antioxidant activity. So, it is believed that people will attach importance to *Eriobotrya* plant for human health.

References

Aytekin, P. A. and Caliskan O. (2007). Loquat production in Turkey. *Acta Horticulturae.* 750:49-53.

Caballere, P. and Fernández, M.A. (2003). Loquat, production and marketing. *Proc. First Int. Loquat Symp. Options Mediterranées* 58:11-20.

Church, C. G.. and Sorber D. G.. (1935). The chemical composition of the loquat. *Fruit Prod. J. Am. Vinegar Ind.* 14:335-340.

De Tommasi, N. (1992b). Constituents of loquat--a study of their antiviral properties. *J. Nat. Prod.* 55:1067-1073.

Dejun, Y. (1979). *The taxonomy of Chinese fruit trees* (ed.). Beijing:Agri. Press. (in Chinese)

Duke, J. and Ayensu, E. S. (1985). *Medicinal plants of China.* Vol. 2. Reference Publ. Algonae, MI. p. 544.

Godoy, H. T. and Rodrigues, A.D. B. (1995), Carotenoid composition and vitamin A value of Brazilian loquat. *Archivos Latinoamericanos Nutrición* 45:336-339.

Hirai, M. (1980). Sugar accumulation and development of loquat fruit. *J, Japan. Soc. Hort. Sci.* 49:347-353.

Huizhi Z., Peng S. A., Cai L. H. et al. (1990). The germplasm resources of the genus *Eriobotrya* with special reference on the origin of *E. japonica* Lindl. *Acta Hort. Sinica* 17: 5-12.

Huxley, A. (1992). *The New Royal Horticultual Society Dictionary of Gardening*(ed.). London: Macmillan.

Ichinose, L. (1995). The origin and development of loquat (in Japanese), *Series of Agr.Tech.* 4 (Supph):l-5.

Kobaa, K., Matsuokab, A., Osadac, K. and Huangd, Y. S. (2007). Effect of loquat (*Eriobotrya japonica*) extracts on LDL oxidation. *Food Chemistry,* 104: 308-316.

Morton. J, F, [ed.]. (1987). Loquat p, 103-108, In: *Fruits of warm climates,* Creative Resource Systems, Winterville. FL.

Noreen, W., Wadood, A., Hidayat,H. K., and Wahid, S A. M. (1988). Effect of loquat on blood glucose levels of normal and alloxan-diabetic rabbits. *Planta Medica,* 54:196-199.

Olaeta, J. A., Undurraga, P. L., Barahona, L. and Feito, X, Y. (2007). Effect of Packaging material and cold storage period on quality of loquat. *Acta Horticulturae.* 750:477-482.

Shaw, P. K. and Wilson, C. W. (1981). Determination of organic acids md sugars in loquat by high-pressure liquid chromatography. *J. Sci. Food Agr.* 32:1242-1246.

Shimizu, M., H., Fukumura, H., Tsuji, S., Tanaami, T. Hayashi, and N. Morita. (1986). Anti-inflamatory constituents of topically applied crude drugs I. Constituents and anti-inflamatory effect of loquat. *Chem. Pharm.. Bul.* 34:2~14-2617.

Shunquan, L., Sharpe R.H, and Janick J. (1999). Loquat: Botany and horticulture. *Hort. Rev.* 23:233-276.

Shunquan, L. (2003). Plant materials in Asian Countries, *Proc. First Int. Loquat Symp. Options Mediterranées*, 58:41-44.

Shunquan, L. (2007). World loquat production and research with special reference to China. *Acta Horticulturae.* 750:43.

Soler, E., Martinez-Calva ,J., Llácer, G., and Badenes, M. L. (2007). Loquat in Spain: Production and Marketing. *Acta Horticulturae.* 750:45-47.

Uchino, K., Tatsuda,Y. and Sakoda, K.. (1994). Relation of harvest date md skin color to fruit quality of loquat 'Magi' during maturation. *J. Japan Soc. Hort. Sci.* 83:479--484.

Xianghui, Y., Glakpe, K., Lin S.Q. et al. (2005). Taxa of plants of genus *Eriobotrya* around the world and native to Southeastern Asia. *J. Fruit Sci.* 22(1):55-60.

Yanping, H., Yanchun, Q., Shunquan, L., Yueming, J., and Feng, C. (2008). Characterization of antioxidant compounds in *Eriobotrya fragrans* Champ.leaf. *Scientia Horticulturae.* 118:288-292.

Yanping, H., Shunquan, L., Yueming, J. and Muhammad, A. (2008). Varation in contents of total phenolics and flavonoids and antioxidant activities in the leaves of 11 Eriobotrya species. *Plant Foods Hum Nutr.* 63:200-204.

Yuexin, Y., Guangya, W., and Xingchang, P. (2002). *China Food Composition, Book1* (eds), Peking: Peking University Medical Press.pp:81-98.

Yonghua, Z., Xi Y. F., and Tiejin, Y. (1993). Studies on post-harvest respiration and ethylene production of loquat fruit. *Acta Hort. Sinica.* 20:111-115.

In: Fruit and Vegetable Consumption and Health
Editors: Anton Papareschi and Harvey Eppolito
ISBN: 978-1-60741-596-1

Chapter VII

Plant Vitamin Antioxidants and Their Influence on the Human Diet

José M. Palma, Francisco J. Corpas and Luis A. del Río
Departamento de Bioquímica, Biología Celular y Molecular de Plantas, Estación Experimental del Zaidín, CSIC, Apartado 419, 18080 Granada, Spain

Abstract

The interest of humans for the diet composition and the link of this concern to a healthy status is growing more and more. Thus, the incorporation of some terms/concepts into our background has greatly improved our knowledge on disciplines such as Nutrition, Dietetics, Physiology and even Biochemistry. In this context, the field of antioxidants has gained special attention due to the involvement of these compounds in the defense against some pathologies and in aging processes. Accordingly, the consumption of antioxidants has notably increased in the first world population as complements of the diet. Some of these antioxidants have a vitamin nature, and the intake of multivitamin additives, either as single or incorporated to the food, has become one of the identities of the consumer society. However, the rule of *the more the better* does not fit in nutrition, and this is obvious. An over-consumption of antioxidants may lead to unexpected effects.

Antioxidants refer to those substances which, in little amounts, are able to prevent the oxidation of other molecules thus avoiding dysfunction of these in the metabolism. These oxidations are mainly promoted by reactive oxygen species (ROS), where oxygen free radicals are included. Plants are the source of many antioxidants with important roles in the human physiology. Thus, vitamin C (ascorbic acid, ascorbate), the paradigm of the antioxidants, is present in plant tissues, fungi and some animal species, but primates are unable to synthesize it. This makes humans be plant-dependent beings at this level. Other major plant antioxidants with vitamin nature include □-tocopherol (vitamin E), □-carotene (provitamin A), and flavonoids. The beneficial role of these compounds in the physiology and in pathological situations and their presence in many natural products have addressed the interest towards the research of many plant species which were always included in our diet but, by some unknown reasons, possibly the present life rhythm, were almost forgotten.

In this chapter, the generation of ROS in biological systems and the role of some plant antioxidants in the scavenging of these ROS will be analyzed. A discussion of how these compounds may influence our diet will be also addressed.

The Oxygen Paradox

Oxygen represents 21% of the atmosphere gases and is a fundamental element for the development of any living system as we know nowadays. The most important reactions in which oxygen takes place include the combustion and the oxidation. In fact, the respiration is the final step of a long combustion process from which we, living beings, obtain energy through burning chemical compounds with high energetic power, basically carbohydrates and lipids. The respiratory pathway resides in the mitochondrial membrane, an organelle considered as the cell energy factory. The respiration process implies that reduced compounds (rich in electrons) become oxidized with the transfer of electrons to oxygen, thus rendering water. This reduction of oxygen to water is basically carried out through four monovalent electronic steps catalyzed by the cytochrome c oxidase, an enzyme immersed in the membrane of mitochondria from eukaryotes organisms. Concomitantly, the energy released in this chemical reaction is accumulated as adenosine triphosphate (ATP), a molecule which is considered as the energetic currency in living beings (Berg et al., 2002).

Alternatively, oxygen is able to participate in diverse chemical reactions where it oxidises other compounds by "sequestering" their electrons. This feature confers to oxygen a great relevance in the aerobic biological systems due to their high surrounding oxygen concentration, and this promotes that biomolecules (nucleic acids, proteins and lipids, among others) may be oxidised, thus losing their specific function. Nowadays, it is well assumed the concept "we age because we are oxidized". In certain sense this assert responses to the fact that the oxidation reactions which normaly take place in our organism are counteracted by defense mechanisms involved in bringing cells to their normal stage. Nevertheless, in pathological situations and during aging in which the organism stops functioning in an optimal condition, oxidation processes gain relevance and notoriousness.

In all reactions, including biochemicals ones, any oxidation process has its own reduction side. Any substance which is oxidised loses an electron and, as a counterpart, another compound is reduced after gaining that electron. Oxygen has the capacity to gain up to four electrons (thus being reduced) is a series of reactions which end with the formation of water (Figure 1). In the transit from oxygen to water three molecules with oxidant power may be formed, some of them having a high reactivity: superoxide radical, hydrogen peroxide, and hydroxyl radical (red color in the scheme of Figure 1). These molecules together with others which share similar reactivity characteristics, formed from oxygen, are collectively called reactive oxygen species (ROS). These ROS include molecules which are free radicals such as superoxide and hydroxyl, which bear an unpaired electron, and non-radicals compounds like hydrogen peroxide, ozone, singlet oxygen, etc. Table 1 summarizes the most common ROS, either radicals or non-radicals.

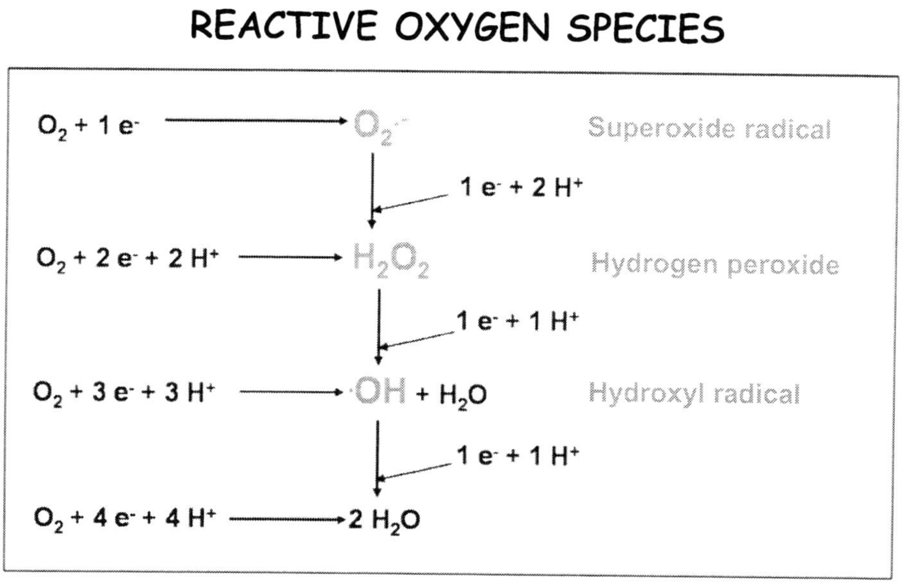

Figure 1. The reduction of oxygen till water is accomplished through four monovalent reactions, in which one electron (1 e^-) per step is transferred. The whole reduction of the oxygen can be also reached in one step through transferring four electrons (Salin 1988). [Reprinted with permission of Ediciones de Horticultura, S.L., Spain].

Table 1. Main reactive oxygen species (ROS)

Radicals	Non radicals
Superoxide ($O_2^{\cdot -}$)	Hyidrogen peroxide (H_2O_2)
Hydroxyl ($^{\cdot}OH$)	Hypoclorous acid (HOCl)
Peroxyl ($RO_2^{\cdot}$)	Ozone (O_3)
Alcoxyl ($RO^{\cdot}$)	Singlet oxygen ($^1O_2$)
Hydroperoxyl ($HO_2^{\cdot}$)	Peroxynitrite ($ONOO^-$)

Summarizing, oxygen, which, as we assert at the beginning of this chapter, is necessary for life, is, conversely, source of high reacting compounds able to alter many biomolecules, thus interfering with their physiological roles in the cell/organism.

ROS Production in Biological Systems

The production of ROS in aerobic cells is not an extraordinary event, since these species are naturally generated in all organisms whose metabolism depends on the oxygen. Thus, from all the oxygen which enters the mitochondria for the respiratory pathway, about 3% is derived to the ROS formation (Raha and Robinson 2000). It could be considered as the "toll" that we have to pay to use the oxygen for our own benefit. Likewise, in chloroplasts, cell organelles where the photosynthesis is carried out, the production of ROS takes place as a consequence of the internal high oxygen concentration. In these cell compartments ROS are generated as secondary by-product of an electron transport chain located in the thylakoids which is responsible for all the photosynthesis light-dependent chemical reactions (Asada, 2006).

Under stress situations or in certain pathologies, cell functioning is altered thus favouring an increase of ROS production. These conditions may promote oxidative stress which, if not avoided, may trigger cell and tissue degradation stages which finally leads to cell death. The cataracts disease easily illustrates this process. The macular degeneration characteristic of cataracts which mostly manifests with aging is promoted by ROS thanks to UV and ionizing radiations (Halliwell and Guteridge 2007). Furthermore, there are other pathologies in human linked to the ROS production. Thus, ROS are involved in diseases such as diabetes, Alzheimer and other neurodegenerative processes and in aging properly (Halliwell and Gutteridge 2007; Seifried et al., 2007). In plants, some cases like those of heavy metal stress, herbicides, high radiation, high and low temperature, ozone excess, drought and salinity, among others, are associated to oxidative stress situations which promote DNA, proteins and lipids alteration. This leads to disorganization of cell membranes and degradation of most cell components (del Río et al., 1999; Smirnoff 2005).

ROS production is not always associated to pathologies. One of the most representative examples of beneficial ROS generation takes place in phagocytes from the blood stream (macrophages and neutrophils). In infectious episodes triggered by bacteria, viruses and pathogens, among others, a superoxide radicals' generation system located in the plasma membrane of phagocytic cells is activated together with a complex phagocytosis process. The generation of superoxide radicals is linked to a marked increase in oxygen uptake in those cells, what has led to call this event as respiratory burst. As indicated by Halliwell and Gutteridge (2007) this is a bad name, since the extra oxygen uptake is not due to an increased respiration and is not prevented by inhibition of mitochondrial electron transport. Under the phagocytosis conditions, the invader organism is engulfed within a phagocytic vacuole or phagosome where distinct ROS are dumped. The engulfed particles are then killed and, if possible, digested within the phagocytic vacuole. For a more detailed illustration of the phagocytosis the reading of the chapter dedicated to this subject is recommended (Halliwell and Gutteridge 2007, pages 405-420).

Likewise, it has been proved that ROS are also essential in some other processes such as the modulation of the immune response. In this case, the dysfunction of the immune system may lead to diseases characterized by inflamatory episodes. In other situations the ROS can function as secondary messengers which favour the activation of specific genes in the response to stimuli linked to cell proliferation and the programmed cell death or apoptosis. These last situations may condition either the tumour extension or that the organism be able to remove the cancerous cells. The list of pathologies where ROS are somehow involved may be enlarged here but, as indicated above, reading of two references already given in this chapter can provide a deeper information for many of them (Halliwell and Gutteridge 2007; Seifried et al., 2007).

Role of Biological Antioxidants

As their own name indicates, antioxidants are compounds able to avoid or prevent the oxidations of distinct molecules of biological interest, thus being oxidized while exerting their role. Chemically what antioxidants do is to scavenge (delete) the capacity of the oxidative substances, specially the ROS, to steel electrons to other molecules. Cells contain the necessary mechanisms to regenerate these antioxidants once they have been oxidized. As a matter of fact, some antioxidants have the capacity to regenerate others in such a way that the initial oxidative effect is buffered in a series of chemical reactions by which the toxic potential of the reactive oxygen species is sequentially diminished. Thus, the function of the antioxidants can be developed either directly by acting over the own ROS, or indirectly by promoting a reducing environment, interfereing with their mechanism, etc. (Smirnoff 2005; Halliwell and Gutteridge 2007).

Classically, the antioxidants have been classified into two groups. On the one hand are those proteins with enzymatic capacity, so they have been called enzymatic antioxidants; on the other hand, the other group includes non-enzymatic antioxidants, which have low molecular weight but not proteic nature. In some case, the non-enzymatic antioxidants correspond to vitamins, so they are strictly necessary for the cell metabolism.

Table 2. Main antioxidative systems reported in plants (Mateos Bernal 2006). Enzymatic antioxidants are those with protein nature. Non-enzymatic antioxidants are small size molecules with non-protein nature.

Enzymatic Antioxidants	Non-enzymatic Antioxidants
Superoxide dismutase	Ascorbic acid, ascorbate (vitamin C)
Catalase	Glutathione
Ascorbate peroxidase	N-acetylcysteine
Monodehydroascorbate reductase	Uric acid
Dehydroascorbate reductase	Glucose
Glutathione reductase	Mannitol
Peroxidases	Albumin
Glutathione S-transferase	α-tocopherol (vitamin E)
Tioredoxins	Carotenoids (provitamin A)
Peroxiredoxins	Flavonoids
Glucose-6-phosphate dehydrogenase	
6-Phosphogluconate dehydrogenase	
Isocitrate dehydrogenase	
Malic enzyme	

In Table 2 the most prominent natural antioxidants are given. Considering all of them, the most interesting, due to the relevance that it is nowadays paid to our diet, are probably the carotenes (provitamin A), ascorbic acid (ascorbate, vitamin C), and α-tocopherol (vitamin E). That is the reason why we will pay more attention to them in the next chapter. Nevertheless, all of them are equally important, since each one has its own specifity against the reactive oxygen species within the diverse cell compartments. Furthermore, the antioxidants do not act independently, as indicated above. They usually are interconnected in a antioxidant network which allows the cell building a global response. Thus, any imbalance among the different antioxidants may trigger a lost of capacity to scavenge and remove the ROS.

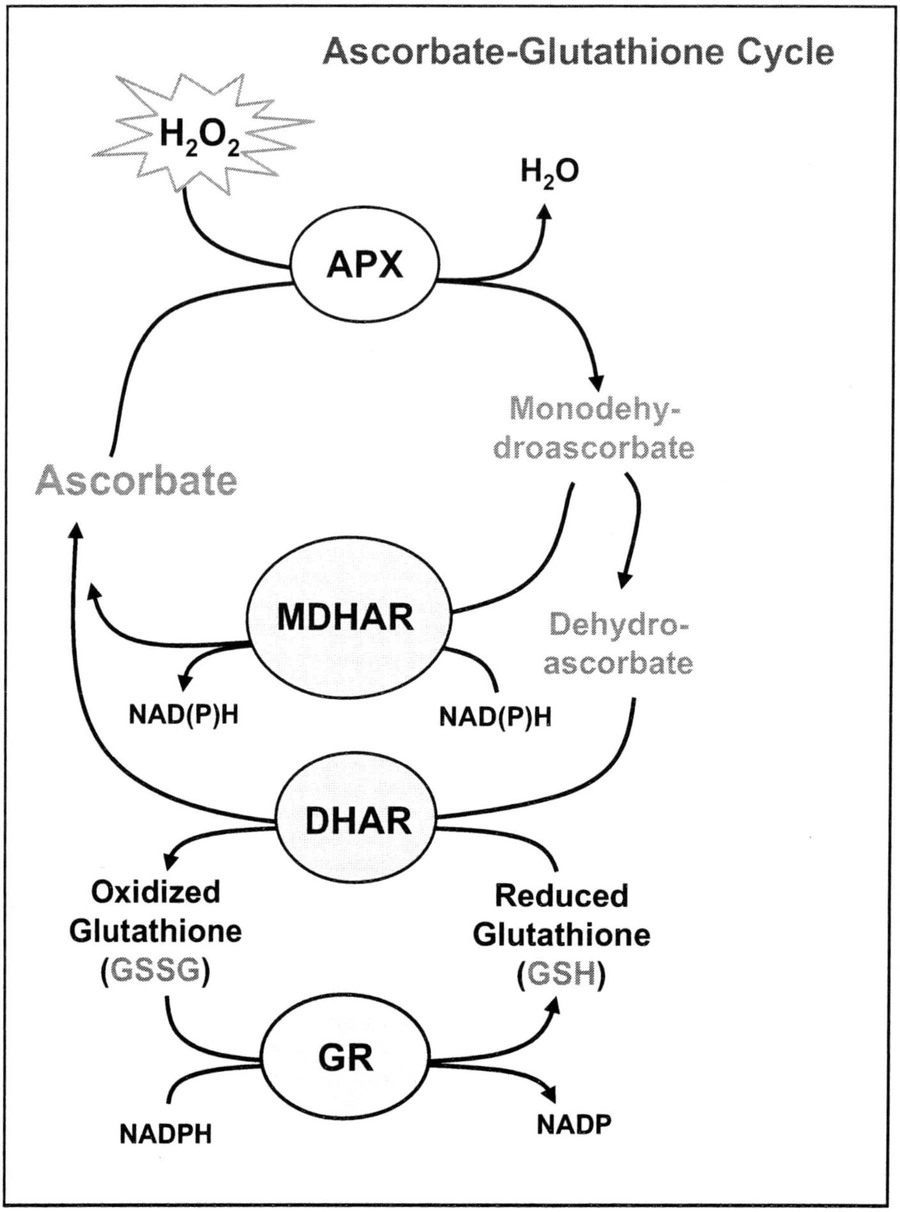

Figure 2. Ascorbate-glutathione cycle reported in higher plants. This cycle also the so called Foyer-Halliwell-Asada pathway integrates four antioxidative enzymes and two non-enzymatic antioxidants. Hydrogen peroxide is decomposed to water by the action of the ascorbate peroxidase, in a process which is lately dependent on the NADPH level. APX, ascorbate peroxidase; MDHAR, monodehydroascorbate reductase; DHAR, dehydroascorbate reductase; GR, glutathione reductase.

As an example, in Figure 2 the ascorbate-glutathione cycle (Asada-Halliwell-Foyer pathway) is depicted. This pathway is exclusive for plants and involves the participation of four enzymatic antioxidants and two small non-enzymatic antioxidants to remove hydrogen peroxide. The enzymes of this pathway are the ascorbate peroxidase (EC 1.11.1.11), the monodehydroascorbate reductase (EC 1.6.5.4), the dehydroascorbate reductase (EC 1.8.5.1), and the glutathione reductase (EC 1.6.4.2). The two small molecules are ascorbate and glutathione, a tripeptide composed by glutamic acid, cysteine and glycin. The different components of this cycle are interconnected in such a way that the hydrogen peroxide is reduced to water and the electrons necessary for this reaction are, at last, provided the NADPH.

Under normal conditions, in the cells there is a balance between the ROS production and their scavenging through the diverse antioxidative systems (Figure 3A). Under certain pathological situations, such as stress or in aging, the balance is altered. In those circumstances, cells suffer metabolic dysfunctions and certain pathways stop functioning in an optimal way and, consequently, an increased ROS production takes place. Moreover, the antioxidative systems are not as effective as in normal conditions: the level of antioxidants is decreased due to the deterioration of the cell metabolism; but in some cases, the antioxidants are modified and cannot carry out their function, thus developing important cell damages promoted by ROS. Under these circumstances, oxidative stress is reached (Figure 2B).

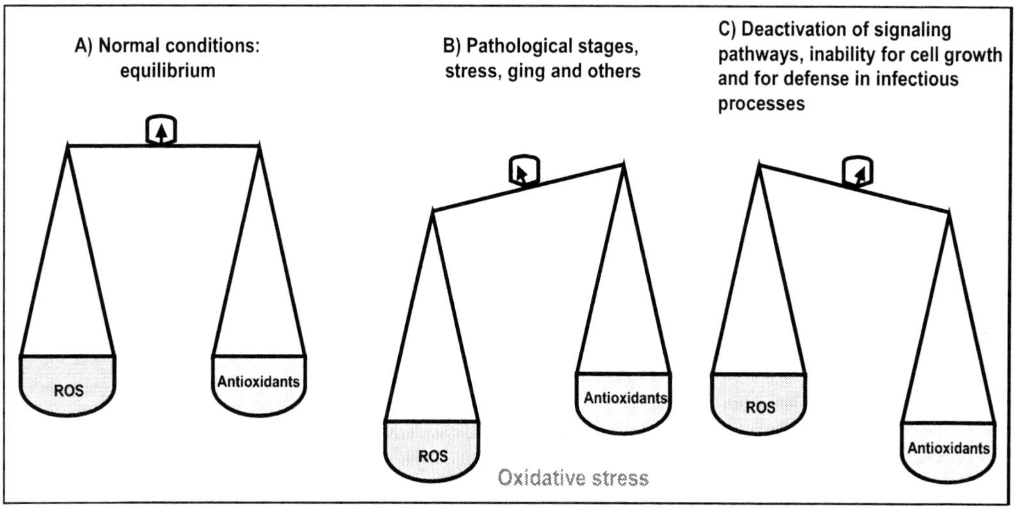

Figure 3. Balance between reactive oxygen species (ROS) and antioxidants under different physiological situations. Under normal equilibrium conditions, antioxidants are able to modulate the internal levels of ROS (A). However, in certain pathological stages, stress and cell aging the ROS production overpass the capacity to scavenge them. In those cases oxidative stress takes place what leads towards cell degeneration processes (B). In most recent studies report that the ROS, besides playing as potent antioxidants, are also involved in signalling mechanisms (transmission of information) triggered in the response against some stimuli. The presence of ROS stimulates the activation of response genes related to cell growth and the defence mechanism in infectious processes. [Reprinted with permission of Ediciones de Horticultura, S.L., Spain].

Antioxidants in the Diet: Vitamins A, C And E

In human beings, the deficiency of the vitamin-type antioxidants (mainly A, C and E) is associated to certain pathologies. In Figure 4 the molecular structure of these vitamins are depicted. Conceptually, vitamins are substances which are required in very little amounts in the diet for the normal dairy functioning of our organism. Vitamin A or retinol represents half of the molecule of the β-carotene (Figure 4). In plants carotenes function as antioxidants due to their ability to quench singlet oxygen and deter its formation during photosynthesis thus avoiding membranes deterioration as a consequence of lipid peroxidation promoted by this ROS (Asada 2006; Halliwell and Gutteridge 2007). This vitamin is essential for growth and cell differentiation, but also for the vision. In fact, vitamin A deficiency is the main cause of the infantile blindness worldwide. It has been proved that, in vitro, carotenoids can diminish the formation of tumours in animals, especially those generated by UVA rays in the skin. Carotenoids are pigments with varying colouring but they are basically red, yellow and orange. Natural products rich in pro-vitamin A carotenoids are tomatoes, carrots, and red peppers, among others, where these compounds are specially accumulated in the plastids. The absence of vitamin A in the diet of the Asian eastern countries, whose main nourishment is based in rice, is origin of the high percentage of pathologies related with the vision deficiency which suffer that geographic region. This hitch has promoted, thanks to a multinational research project financed by public funding, the generation of transgenic strains of golden rice rich in carotenes (http://www.goldenrice.org/).

Vitamin E or α-tocopherol (Figure 4) is fundamental for the structural maintenance of the biological membranes. In studies carried out in the laboratory it has been proved that, in animals, the inclusion of vitamin E in the diet is essential for the maintenance of a number of functions. Due to its lipophylic nature, vitamin E is easily integrated within the biological membranes. As a matter of fact, thylakoids are chloroplastic membrane structures highly rich in α-tocopherol. Vitamin E is a antioxidant due to its capacity to directly quench singlet oxygen, which due to its physico-chemical properties easily attacks lipidic structures. The main sources of vitamin can be found in wheat germ, plant oils, margarines, nuts, seeds and green leaves (Halliwell and Gutteridge, 2007). The absence of vitamin E in the diet does not cause any defficiency pathology in short time, although in premature babies low levels of vitamin E may predispose to those who are affected to develop haemolytic anemia.

Moreover, it has been described a number of dysfunctions associated to low levels of vitamin, although, at present, this field is been thoroughly investigated.

Epidemiological studies suggest that vitamin C plays an important role in the prevention of cardiovascular diseases, especially those which involve an endothelial dysfunction (Kris-Etherton et al., 2004). Vitamin C (Figure 4) is a potent antioxidant derived from glucose throughout a multi-step biosynthetic pathway. Besides its capacity to directly scavenge several ROS, ascorbate is able to regenerate other antioxidants previously oxididised such as carotenoids and vitamin E, what confers to vitamin C a double power. The vitamin C deficiency give rise to scurvy, a disease known centuries ago, since it affected sailors in large crossings. In natural products, the highest contents of vitamin C are detected in pepper, either green, red or yellow, kiwi, strawberry, broccoli, citrics and others (Proteggente et al 2002; Mateos Bernal 2006). Considering all these products, pepper is one of the vegetable which contains the greatest amount on vitamin C per fresh weight, in spite of that are citrics the products which erroneously are considered as the main store of this vitamin. In fact, 0.1% of the pepper fresh weight corresponds to ascorbic acid. The amount of vitamin C in this vegetable is such that about 80 g (1/4 of a California-type pepper fruits) would be enough to satisfy our vitamin diary needs (Mateos Bernal 2006).

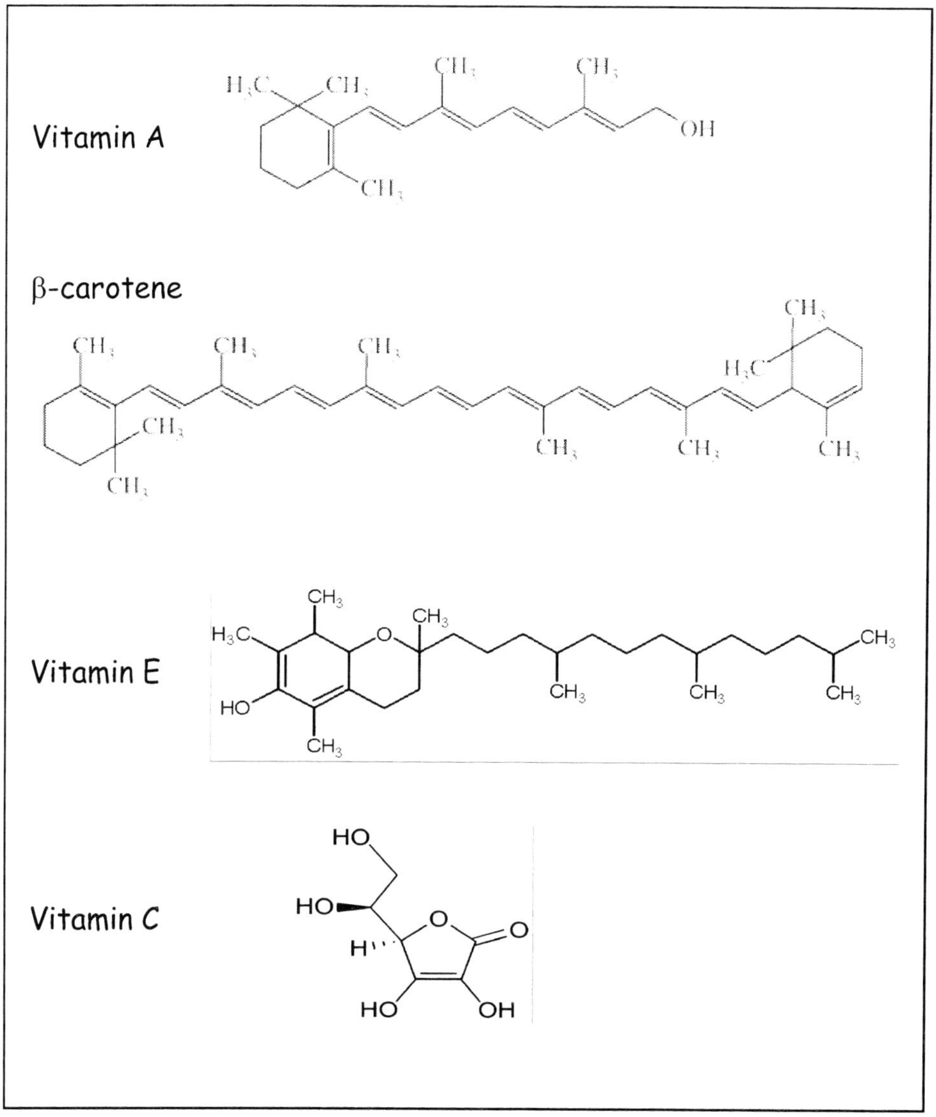

Figure 4. Molecular structure of vitamins A, E and C.

All primates, including humans, have lost the capacity to synthesize vitamin C what makes us almost strictly dependent of the plant kingdom for its obtaining. Thus, unlike other animals, human lacks the presence of the last enzyme of the ascorbate biosynthetic pathway, the gulono-lactone oxidase. This enzyme in plants is slightly different, since uses as substrate the galactono-lactone which is converted to ascorbic acid through a galactono-lactone dehydrogenase activity. Thus, due to its metabolic singularity, the search and availability of vitamin C-enriched sources is essential for our diet. One of the most interesting questions which concerns to pepper biochemistry/physiology nowadays is the role of ascorbic acid in this plant species, basically to such huge amount found in fruits. Among the hypotheses which have been raised, one of them proposes that ascorbate functions as a redox buffer in the plant physiology (Palma et al., 2007), a role which was also proposed earlier for this vitamin in plant cells (Foyer and Noctor 2005).

In situations of vitaminic starving it is, in general, recommended the oral administration of vitaminic complexes to compensate the deficit. At present, we are in a situation in which, according to the USA Nutritional Service and National Health, more than half of the population intakes dietetic supplements, one third multivitaminic complexes, and one eighth uses supplements of vitamin E and/or C (Seifried et al., 2007). If there is not deficit, the intake of vitaminic complexes overloads the organism with substances which, as a matter of fact, would be unnecessary. The present life style and the unknowledge of all metabolic concerns of the ROS and the antioxidants have made that, in a non discriminatory way, we human beings from the first world have been converted into vitamin sinks. Once proved the benefits of the antioxidants, our society postulated the idea of *the more the better*. And this, like in other aspects related to nutrition, is a false assertion.

Conclusions: Are Antioxidants Good?

In the previous chapters we have brought light to some of the concepts and involvements referred to the ROS and the antioxidants. We have given some examples on the beneficial effects of both. Besides, there is not doubt that, according to our present knowledge of the state of the art, an excess of either ROS or antioxidants may be pernicious. However, this concept can be also attributed to any other food, regardless the nutritional excelences that it might have. An overproduction of ROS promotes oxidative stress which results in episodes of programmed cell death, cancer and other pathologies. On the contrary, an overload of antioxidants (Figure 3C) would contribute to reduce the levels of necessary ROS – useful as signaling molecules transmitting information – of a number of cell respones in situations such as cancer and those where the immune system is involved.

As asserted by Halliwel and Gutteridge (2007) in their very recommendable handbook, "…the evidence supporting an antioxidant role for carotenoids in animals is weak. However, this does not mean they are unimportant; they could exert beneficial effects by other mechanisms, regulating cell-cell communication or gene expression…" What is clear is that antioxidants are a promising therapy for the prevention and the treatment of certain diseases. Thus, it has been proved the existence of a correlation between a diet rich in fruits and vegetables and a lower risk to develop cancer and cardivascular diseases (Seifried et al., 2007). Likewise, during the menopausic episodes, the favourable effects of the antioxidant from the diet have been reported (Miquel et al 2006). Similarly, we could continue describing a plethora of the beneficial effects which have been registered in thousands of scientific publications. Summarizing, what it has been consensed on the behalf of all specialists is that a diet rich in fruits and vegetables (Figure 5) promotes a higher health status and, therefore, the increase in the life quality. It is always preferable consuming a natural product rather than a manufactured one or a pill enriched in many compounds which not always are sinergic with our metabolism (Halliwell 1999; Bonnefoy et al 2002).

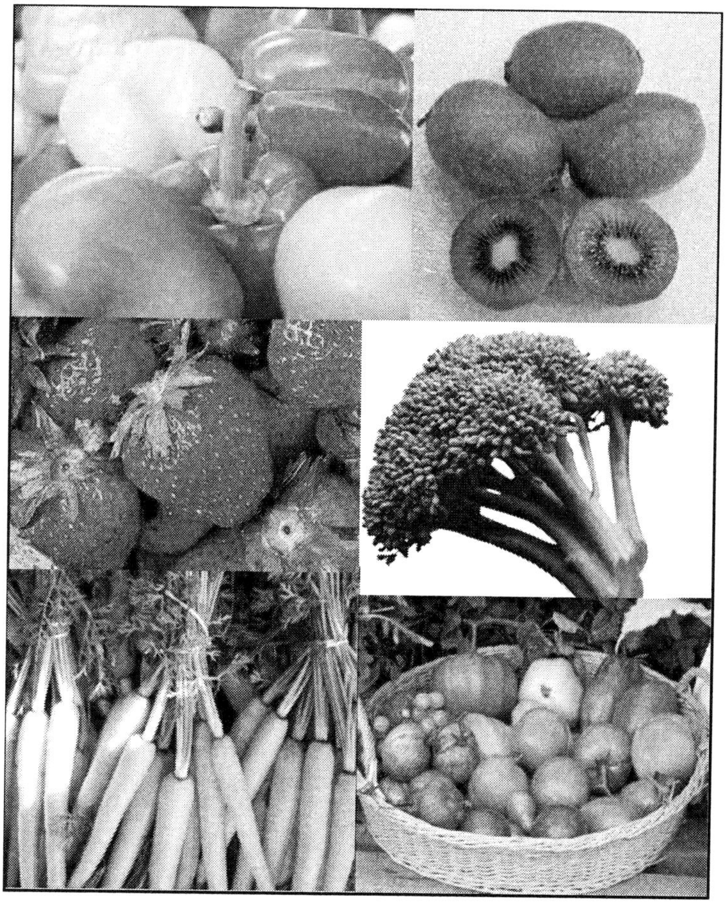

Figure 5.

As the last conclusion we could go back again to the concept of equilibrium (balance). And nothing more appropriate that the image of the Man of Vitrubio, that design by Leonardo da Vinci who, long time ago, showed the sense of proportions in nature and, consequently, of the man within the environment. As we always recommend, vitamins, as well as other antioxidants, have to be always taken in the right extent/way (Palma and del Río 2006).

Acknowledgement

Authors are grateful for the financial support of their research on antioxidants to projects from the Ministry of Education and Science (AGL2005-00101 and BIO2006-14949-C02-02) and Junta de Andalucía (P06-CVI-1820), Spain.

Bibliography

Asada K (2006). Production and scavenging of reactive oxygen species in chloroplasts and their functions. *Plant Physiol.* 141: 391-396.

Bonnefoy M, Drai J, Kostka T (2002) Antioxidants to slow aging, facts and perspectives. *Presse Médique* 31: 1174-1184.

Berg JM, Tymoczko JL, Stryer L (2002) Biochemistry, 5th edition. Freeman, **ISBN:** 0716746840.

Foyer CH, Noctor G (2005) Redox homeostasis and antioxidant signalling: a metabolic interface between stress perception and physiological responses.*Plant Cell* 17: 1866-1875.

Halliwell B (1999) Vitamin C: poison, prophylactic or panacea? Trends in Biochemical Science 24: 255-259.

Halliwell B, Gutteridge JMC (2007) Free *Radicals in Biology and Medicine.* Oxford University Press, Oxford.

Kris-Etherton PM, Lichtenstein AH, Howard BV, Steinberg D, Wiztum JL, Nutrition Committee of the American Heart Association Council on Nutrition, Physical Activity, Metabolism (2004) Antioxidant vitamin supplements and cardiovascular disease. *Circulation* 110, 637-641.

Miquel J, Ramírez-Boscá A, Ramírez-Boscá JV, Alperi JD (2006) Menopuase: a review on the role of oxygen stress and favorable effects of dietary antioxidants. *Archives of Gerontology and Geriatrics* 42, 289-306.

Mateos Bernal RM (2006) Antioxidantes de pimiento (Capsicum annuum L.): Estudio Bioquím. O y molecular de la maduración del fruto y de la respuesta a estrés abiótico. Tesis Doctoral, Universidad de Granada.

Palma JM, Mateos RM, Jiménez A, Corpas FJ, Sevilla S, del Río LA (2007) Role of the ascorbate in the physiology of the pepper fruit (*Capsicum annuum* L.). VIII Reunión del Grupo Español de Radicales Libres, Abstract Book, Valencia, Spain.

Proteggente AR, Pannala AS, Paganga G, Van Buren L, Wagner E, Wiseman S, Van De Put F, Dacombe C, Rice-Evans CA (2002) The antioxidant activity of regularly consumed fruit and vegetables reflects their phenolic and vitamin C composition. *Free Radical Research* 36, 217-233.

Raha S, Robinson BH (2000) Mitochondria, oxygen free radicals, disease and ageing. *Trends Biochem. Sci.* 25: 502-508.

del Río LA, Palma JM, Sandalio LM, Navari-Izzo F (1999) *Free Radical Research* 31, Suppl., 1-256.

Salin ML (1988) Toxic oxygen species and protective systems of the chloroplast. *Physiologia Plantarum* 72, 681-689.

Seifried HE, Anderson DE, Fisher EI, Milner JA (2007) A review of the interaction among dietary antioxidants and reactive oxygen species. *Journal of Nutritional Biochemistry*, DOI 10.1016/j.jnutbio.2006.10.007.

Smirnoff N (2005) *Antioxidants and Reactive Oxygen Species in Plants.* Blackwell Publishing Ltd, Oxford.

In: Fruit and Vegetable Consumption and Health
Editors: Anton Papareschi and Harvey Eppolito

ISBN: 978-1-60741-596-1

Chapter VIII

Kids Choice Program Improves Two Weight Management Behaviors in School Children

Helen M. Hendy[a*], *Keith E. Williams*[b], *Thomas S. Camise*[c], *Deirdre Rahn*[a], *Courtney Costigan*[a], *Scott Gaskins*[a] *and Christina Moyer*[a]
[a]Psychology Program, Penn State University, Schuylkill Campus, PA, USA
[b]Feeding Program, Pediatrics, Penn State Hershey Medical Center, Hershey, PA, USA
[c]Schuylkill Haven Area School District, Schuylkill Haven, PA, USA

Abstract

The Kids Choice Program (Hendy, Williams, and Camise, 2005) was designed as a school-based program to increase children's weight management behaviors while in their everyday environments and while in the company of their peers. The present application of the program targeted two weight management behaviors: eating fruits and vegetables first during the meal (FVFIRST), choosing low-fat and low-sugar healthy drinks (HDRINK). Lunch observations revealed that 82 intervention-group children showed more improvements in both FVFIRST and HDRINK than did 85 control-group children. The Kids Choice Program shows promise for long-term adoption by schools because it is simple in design (children wear nametags, stars are punched into nametags when children choose healthy behaviors, weekly Reward Days let children trade stars for small prizes), because it is relatively low in cost ($2 per child per month of application), and because it is well-accepted by children and their parents.

Keywords: child obesity, weight management, Kids Choice Program

* Author for correspondence: Helen M. Hendy, Ph.D., Psychology Program, Penn State University, Schuylkill Campus, 200 University Drive, Schuylkill Haven, PA, 17972; phone: (570) 385-6069, fax: (570) 385-6135, email: HL4@PSU.EDU.

Introduction

Recent reviews document the effectiveness of school-based programs to improve weight management behaviors in children, with consumption of fruits and vegetables (FV) most often selected as the target behavior (Blanchette and Brug, 2005; Howerton et al., 2007; Knai, Pomerlau, Lock, and McKee, 2006). Many of these programs require multiple components that may include teachers adding nutrition curriculum, cafeteria staff modifying food lunch, cafeteria aides monitoring and rewarding children's food choices, nurses organizing special health presentations, office staff making loudspeaker announcements, and parents completing health activities with their children at home. Unfortunately, improvements seen in children's weight management behavior typically last only as long as the programs are in place. More long-term adoption by schools would certainly be influenced by the program's cost and acceptability (Baranowski et al., 2000; Bauer, Yang, and Austin, 2004; Perry et al., 1998; Reynolds et al., 2000), but little research documents program costs or acceptability ratings from children and their parents. We believe the ideal school-based program for long-term adoption would be one that could be demonstrated to be effective for improving children's weight management behaviors, simple in design, low in cost, and high in acceptability.

The Kids Choice Program was developed as a school-based intervention to improve children's weight management behaviors in their everyday environments. The first application of the program focused on children's FV consumption (Hendy, Williams, and Camise, 2005), which showed improvements that lasted thoughout the one-month intervention, and both for average-weight and overweight children within the sample (Hendy, Williams, Camise, Alderman, Ivy, and Reed, 2007). The Kids Choice Program includes three simple school procedures: (1) Children wear nametags during school lunch with their classmates. (2) Star-shaped holes are punched into the nametags when children show specific small amounts of the targeted weight management behaviors, with at least two choices being available for each behavior. (3) Reward Days are presented once each week for children to trade their stars for small prizes. The procedures of the Kids Choice Program procedures were chosen for a number of reasons. For example, the small and delayed rewards (with stars given daily as token reinforcement, but with prizes available only once a week as back-up reinforcement) were chosen to remove the daily focus from prizes so that children have an opportunity to discover pleasing properties of the weight management behaviors themselves (Hitt, Marriott, and Esser, 1992). The availability of at least two choices for each target behavior was chosen to reduce the risk of satiation effects (Rolls, Rolls, Rowe, and Sweeney, 1981), as were the small daily expectations for each behavior (such as requiring that children eat only 1/8 cup of FV to earn a star). Small daily expectations were also chosen so children could gradually accumulate the repeated taste experiences that appear necessary to learn to enjoy a new food (Birch and Marlin, 1982; Wardle, Herrera, Cooke, and Gibson, 2003). Finally, the presentation of the program during school lunch was chosen to make incidental peer modeling available for the target behaviors, which may be even more powerful than the use of trained peer models (Hendy, 2002; Hendy and Raudenbush, 2000).

One purpose of the present study was to examine the effectiveness of the Kids Choice Program for increasing two weight management behaviors not included in the original study:

(1) FVFIRST = Eating FV first during meals, which may serve as a portion control strategy because it reduces mealtime calorie consumption in adults by up to 12% (Rolls, Roe, and Meeng, 2004). Eating FV first during meals may also enhance the palatability and acceptance of the FV because they would then be eaten when children are most hungry. (2) HDRINK = Choosing healthy drinks that are low-fat and low-sugar, which may reduce the total calories that children consume during meals (CDCP, 2000). Another purpose of the present study was to evaluate the potential of the Kids Choice Program for long-term application in schools by measuring its cost per child and its acceptability ratings by children and their parents.

Methods

Participants

The primary participants of the present study were elementary school children for whom the Kids Choice Program was presented during school lunch, for whom lunch observations were conducted, and for whom statistical analyses examined changes in the two weight management behaviors (FVFIRST, HDRINK) from baseline conditions through a one-month intervention. The study was conducted with 320 1st to 3rd grade children from a school in a small town in Pennsylvania, but in a different school district than the school sampled in the original study (165 boys, 155 girls; 90 first graders, 116 second graders, 114 third graders; mean age = 7.9 years, SD = 1.0; over 95% Caucasian). Of the total 320 children, 167 (52.2%) children usually ate the school-provided lunch and the present study focused on their changes in weight management behaviors (93 boys, 74 girls; mean age = 8.1 years, SD = 0.9; 38 first graders, 65 second graders, 64 third graders; with 85 randomly assigned to the control group and 82 to the intervention group as described below). The remaining 153 children usually brought home-packed lunches, and because of the extreme variability of foods available in these lunches and the difficulty of reliably recording foods eaten from sacks and boxes (Simons-Morton et al., 1992), consumption of home-packed lunches was not included in analyses of the present study. However, so that children bringing home-packed lunches would not feel left out, they wore nametags and received stars for their behaviors as did children eating the school-provided lunch.

Other study participants included children and parents who provided acceptability ratings for the Kids Choice Program two weeks after completion of the intervention phase of the study. Of the total 320 children, parents of 199 (62.2%) children gave permission for child interviews used to gather children's program acceptability ratings, with a random subset of 154 (77.4%) of these children chosen because of limits of time and interviewer availability (73 boys, 81 girls; mean age = 8.0 years, SD = 1.0; 35 first graders, 55 second graders, 64 third graders; with 81 children from the control group and 73 from the intervention group). Of the 199 parents who gave permission for child interviews, 151 (75.9%) parents also returned brief questionnaires to provide their own program acceptability ratings (with their children including 69 boys, 82 girls; mean age = 7.9 years, SD = 0.9; 41 first graders, 60 second graders, 50 third graders; with 85 children from the control group and 66 from the intervention group).

School lunch observations

To evaluate changes in the children's two weight management behaviors (FVFIRST, HDRINK) from baseline conditions through intervention conditions, 10 advanced Psychology undergraduates were trained as lunch observers. Inter-observer reliability trials were conducted with observers using a prepared datasheet to record FVFIRST and HDRINK behaviors for 14 adult volunteers who simulated "children" at school lunch, with the mean agreement score found to be 92% for FVFIRST and 100% for HDRINK.

School lunch observations during baseline conditions were conducted three days a week for two weeks, with the first week used to habituate children to the presence of observers. Children wore nametag necklaces in a variety of neon-colors and in the shape of a cat's pawprint. Observers stood quietly at the side of the lunch tables with their prepared datasheets during the first 10 minutes of the 30 minute lunch period. First they recorded the names of up to 14 children seated in their observation area. Then they recorded the time-sensitive behavior of FVFIRST, defined as the child eating at least 1/8 cup of fruit or vegetable first during the meal. Finally, they recorded the behavior of HDRINK, defined as the child choosing a low-fat and low-sugar beverage for lunch. The school-provided lunch always included at least two FV choices and at least two HDRINK choices. (NOTE: To avoid inflated FVFIRST scores, potato foods were not considered vegetables for the present study. Also, because the opaque beverage cartons used by the school made it difficult to determine the exact amount of fluid consumed, HDRINK was measured only as the type of drink chosen by the child while in the lunch line. However, we have observed that nearly 100% of children open and drink from their chosen cartons.)

School lunch observations during intervention conditions were conducted three days a week for four weeks. A random half of the children from each classroom were assigned to the "LIONS" intervention group. These intervention-group children were told they could earn stars punched into their nametags by choosing "Good Health Behaviors" that included eating "about four big bites" (about 1/8 cup) of FV first during the meal (FVFIRST), and choosing a low-fat and low-sugar healthy drink such as 1% or 2% white milk, water, or 100% fruit juice (HDRINK). The other half of the children were assigned to the "TIGERS" control group and told they could earn stars by choosing "Good Citizenship Behaviors" that included talking quietly during lunch and keeping their lunch area clean. Children's group assignments were indicated by small letters on the back of their nametags to help them remember which behaviors earned them stars. Children were also told that once a week they would have a Reward Day during lunch when they could trade five stars for one small prize.

To reduce the risk of observer expectation effects during intervention conditions that could distort their records of children's behavior according to group assignment, a two-part lunchtime procedure was used to disconnect the observers' records of children's behaviors from the delivery of stars punched into children's nametags. Part one took place in the first 10 minutes of the 30 minute lunch period, during which the observers used their datasheets to record each child's name, FVFIRST behavior, HDRINK behavior, and to note any reprimands received from school staff for talking too loudly or making a mess. Part two took place in the last 10 minutes of the 30 minute lunch period, during which the observers walked down the lunch tables with completed datasheets to deliver stars to children according to their group assignment as shown on the back of their nametags.

Reward Days were presented once each week to give children the opportunity to trade their stars for small prizes (e.g., Playdoh, notebooks, fancy pencils, gliders, water bottles, puzzles, stuffed animals, silly hats). A large table was set up in the corner of the lunch room with large plastic bins containing a selection of five or six prizes. Research assistants punched a special code into children's nametags once they traded their stars for prizes, and children were allowed to save any leftover stars until the next Reward Day.

Program acceptability ratings

To gather acceptability ratings from the children two weeks after the Kids Choice Program intervention, individual child interviews were conducted (n = 154). The interviews were conducted by trained interviewers who used a prepared interview script and who were kept blind as to the children's earlier assignment to intervention or control groups. To reduce the probability that children would inflate their ratings in hopes of receiving rewards, children were reminded that the Kids Choice Program was finished and no more stars or prizes would be given. Each child was called into the hallway just outside the cafeteria and given a laminated card with three cartoon faces (frown, neutral, smile). To gather three-point acceptability ratings, children were asked to point to the face that showed how much they liked the Kids Choice Program that was brought to their school (with the frown = 1, neutral face = 2, smile = 3).

To gather acceptability ratings from parents two weeks after the Kids Choice Program intervention, brief questionnaires were completed by parents (n = 151) using a five-point scale (from 1 = not at all to 5 = very) for how acceptable the Kids Choice Program would be "as an ongoing program done throughout the school year."

Results

Changes in children's weight management behaviors

To examine the effectiveness of the Kids Choice Program for increasing the two weight management behaviors shown by children during school lunch (FVFIRST, HDRINK), 3 X 2 repeated-measures ANOVAs were used with three study phases serving as the within-subjects factor (one three-meal block under baseline conditions, two three-meal blocks under intervention conditions), and with the two study groups serving as the between-subjects factor (n = 82 in the intervention group rewarded for "Good Health Behaviors," n = 85 in the control group rewarded for "Good Citizenship Behaviors"). FVFIRST was measured as the number of meals in the three-meal-block for which the child ate 1/8 cup of FV first during the meal. HDRINK was measured as the number of meals in the three-meal-block for which the child chose a low-fat and low-sugar healthy drink. (NOTE: A total of 12 intervention meals were observed, but to avoid losing children from the analyses because they were absent or brought home-packed lunches for some of these meals, each child's score for FVFIRST and HDRINK was defined as the number of meals the behavior occurred for the first six recorded intervention meals, divided into three three-meal-blocks.) If the KCP was effective for increasing the weight management behaviors, we anticipated that these ANOVAs would find a significant interaction between study phase and study group, with the intervention and control groups showing similar behavior under baseline conditions, but with the intervention group showing more of the behavior under intervention conditions.

Results indicated that both FVFIRST and HDRINK weight management behaviors increased with the application of the Kids Choice Program. For FVFIRST (Figure 1a), a significant interaction was found between study phase and study group ($F_{(2,330)} = 7.81$, $p < .001$) with post-hoc comparisons showing no difference between intervention and control groups for FVFIRST in baseline ($t_{(165)} = 1.28$, $p < .21$), but significantly more FVFIRST by the intervention group after three meals of intervention ($t_{(165)} = 3.60$, $p < .001$) and after six meals of intervention ($t_{(165)} = 4.44$, $p < .001$). The changes in FVFIRST shown by the 82 intervention-group children revealed a partial Eta^2 effect size = .50.

Similarly for HDRINK (Figure 1b), a significant interaction was found between study phase and study group ($F_{(2,330)} = 20.35$, $p < .001$), with post-hoc comparisons showing no difference between intervention and control groups for HDRINK in baseline ($t_{(165)} = .45$, $p < .66$), but significantly more HDRINK by the intervention group after three meals of intervention ($t_{(165)} = 4.39$, $p < .001$) and after six meals of intervention ($t_{(165)} = 6.27$, $p < .001$). The changes in HDRINK shown by the 82 intervention-group children revealed a partial Eta^2 effect size = .63.

Kids Choice Program cost and acceptability

The nametag necklaces children wore during lunch could be easily produced with supplies already on hand at the school. The primary expense of the Kids Choice Program was then the small prizes offered during the weekly Reward Days, when children could trade in "stars" in their nametags they had earned for their behavior choices. The cost of these small prizes was approximately $2 per child per month of application of the Kids Choice Program. The 154 children interviewed gave a mean acceptability rating for the Kids Choice Program of 2.9 ($SD = 0.3$) using their three-point scale, and the 151 parents who completed brief questionnaires gave a mean acceptability rating of 4.4 ($SD = 0.9$) using their five-point scale.

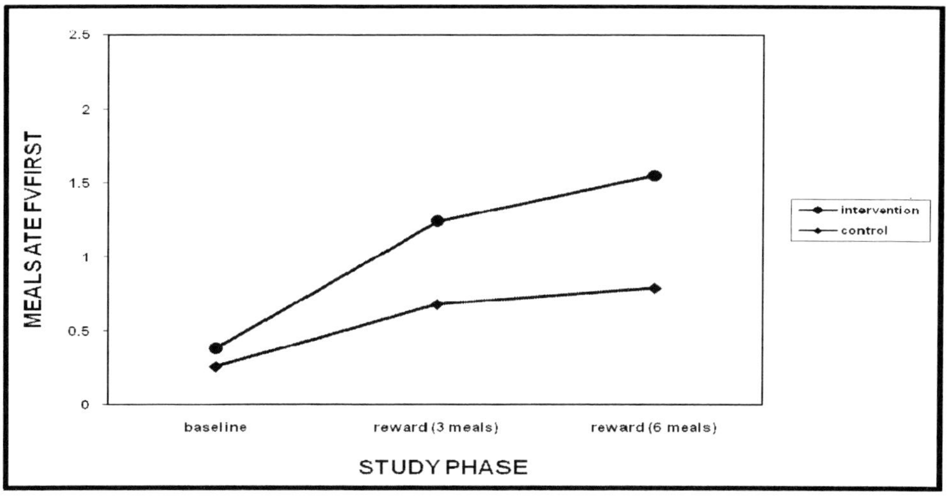

Figure 1a.

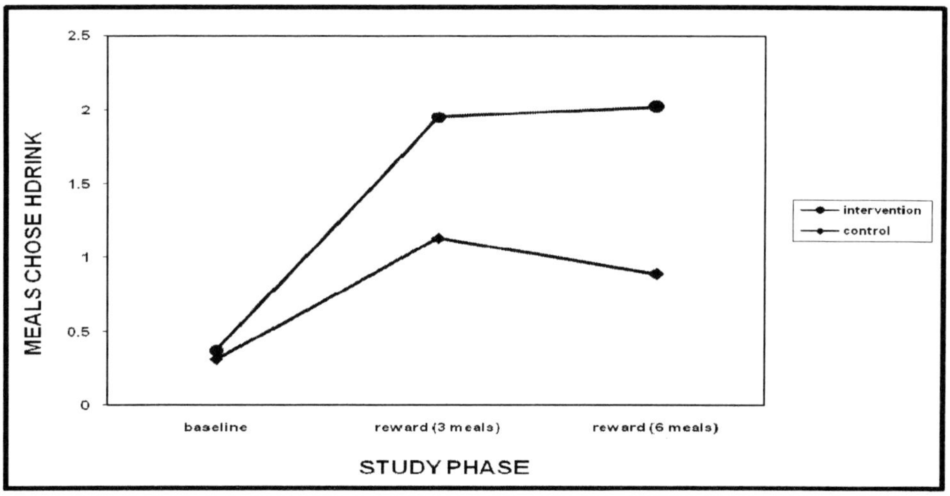

Figure 1b.

Figure 1. Changes in two weight management behaviors (FVFIRST, HDRINK) for children in two study groups (intervention, control) across three study phases (one three-meal-block under baseline, two three-meal-blocks under reward intervention). Children in the intervention group ($\underline{n} = 82$) received rewards for "Good Health Behaviors" that included eating FV first during school lunch (FVFIRST) and choosing a low-fat and low-sugar healthy drink (HDRINK). Children in the control group ($\underline{n} = 85$) received rewards for "Good Citizenship Behaviors" that included talking quietly and keeping their lunch area clean. **(a)** Changes in the number of meals children in each study group ate FVFIRST across the three study phases. Repeated-measures ANOVA found a significant interaction between study phase and study group ($\underline{p} < .001$), with paired comparisons showing no group difference in baseline, but more FVFIRST for the intervention group after three meals and six meals of reward intervention. **(b)** Changes in the number of meals children in each study group chose HDRINK across the three study phases. Repeated-measures ANOVA found a significant interaction between study phase and study group ($\underline{p} < .001$), with paired comparisons showing no group difference in baseline, but more HDRINK for the intervention groups after three meals and six meals of reward intervention.

Discussion

The present study demonstrated that the Kids Choice Program was effective for increasing two recommended weight management behaviors for school children (CDCP, 2000): Eating FV first during the meal (FVFIRST), and choosing low-fat and low-sugar healthy drinks (HDRINK). The present results replicate findings from the first application of the Kids Choice Program (Hendy, Williams, and Camise, 2005), which found the program effective for increasing FV consumption (with FV eaten anytime during the meal) for both average-weight and overweight children (Hendy et al., 2007). We believe the Kids Choice Program shows promise for long-term adoption by schools for a number of reasons: (1) The program is simple in design with children wearing nametag necklaces during school lunch, with stars punched into nametags when children choose healthy behaviors, and with Reward Days presented once a week for children to trade their stars for small prizes. Although college sudent research assistants delivered the stars to children's nametags in the present evaluation of the program, one 15-minute session could be used to train school staff or parent volunteers to perform the same role. (2) The program is relatively low in cost at $2 per child per month of application. The nametag necklaces can be made with available school supplies, and the small prizes are available in bulk from a variety of vendors. Costs may be reduced further by community-donated prizes, by Parent Teacher Organization fund-drives, or by applications for state-sponsored wellness grants. (3) The program receives excellent acceptability ratings from children and parents.

One limitation of the present study was that lunch observers were not blind to the children's group assignment because they later delivered stars to the children according to their group assignments coded on their nametags. However, we believe that any observer expectation effects were minimal or absent in the present results showing that the Kids Choice Program increased children's FVFIRST and HDRINK behaviors during school lunch. The fast pace and intense concentration required of observers during the first 10 minutes of lunch when they recorded the children's behaviors gave them little time to think about the children's group assignments until the last 10 minutes of lunch, when they looked at the coded nametags in order to deliver the children's earned stars. In addition, the strong interobserver reliability scores demonstrated by lunch observers for the FVFIRST and HDRINK behaviors (92% and 100%, respectively) suggest that they were working with very clear definitions for these behavioral outcome measures.

Another limitation of the present study was that it was conducted with a sample of mostly Caucasian children from a small town in Pennsylvania. Future research could investigate the effectiveness of the Kids Choice Program for a more ethnically and regionally diverse sample of children. In addition, the present analysis of the Kids Choice Program was applied to only two weight management behaviors (FVFIRST, HDRINK) that did not include exercise, another highly recommended weight management behavior for children (CDCP, 2000). Also, the present application of the progrm was for only four weeks, which was not long enough to expect the program to improve children's weight status. Future research could extend the application of the Kids Choice Program to all three recommended weight management behaviors (FVFIRST, HDRINK, EXERCISE) and present it for a longer period of time to examine whether the program could improve not only the children's weight management behaviors, but also their weight status. Finally, future research could investigate the acceptability of the various components of the Kids Choice Program to school staff, such as their ratings for each of the possible weight management behaviors to be targeted, the nametags worn by children, the timing and location of Reward Days, and the individuals who might best deliver the program to children (e.g., school staff, parent volunteers, older children, college students).

Acknowledgments

The research was supported by grants from Penn State University. We also thank Jennifer Cinelli, Cory Commings, Patricia Denchy, Jeremy Eltringham, Koren Frey, Marc Gabardi, Taryn Huey, Lisa Karavage, Conny Kluegling, Cobi Michael, Lisa Moyer, Matthew Parsley, Harry Pytak, and Kira Wertz.

References

Baranowski, T., Davis, M., Resnicow, K., Baranowski, J., Doyle, C., Lin, L. S., Smith, M., and Wang, D. T. (2000). Gimme-5 fruit, juice and vegetables for fun and health: Outcome evaluation. *Health Education and Behavior, 27,* 96-111.

Bauer, K. W., Yang, Y. W., and Austin, S. B. (2004). "How can we stay healthy when you're throwing all of this in front of use?" Findings from focus groups and interviews in middle schools on environmental influences on nutrition and physical activity. *Health Education and Behavior, 31,* 34-36.

Birch, L. L., and Marlin, D. W. (1982). I don't like it; I never tried it. Effects of exposure on two-year-old children's food preference. *Appetite, 3,* 353-360.

Blanchette L., and Brug, J. (2005). Determinants of fruit and vegetable consumption among 6-12-year old children and effective interventions to increase consumption. *Journal of Human Nutrition and Diet, 18,* 431-43.

Centers for Disease Control and Prevention. (2000). *School health index for physical activity and health eating: A self-assessment and planning guide.* Atlanta, GA: Author.

Hendy, H. M. (2002). Effectiveness of trained peer models to encourage food acceptance in preschool children. *Appetite, 39,* 217-225.

Hendy, H. M., and Raudenbush, B. (2000). Effectiveness of teacher modeling to encourage food acceptance in preschool children. *Appetite, 34,* 61-76.

Hendy, H. M., Williams, K. E., and Camise, T. S. (2005). "Kids Choice" school program increases children's fruit and vegetable acceptance. *Appetite, 45,* 250-263.

Hendy, H. M., Williams, K. E., Camise, T. S., Alderman, S., Ivy, J., and Reed, J. (2007). Overweight and average-weight children equally responsive to "Kids Choice Program" to increase fruit and vegetable consumption. *Appetite, 49,* 683-686.

Hitt, D. D., Marriott, R. G., and Esser, J. K. (1992). Effects of delayed rewards and task interest on intrinsic motivation. *Basic and Applied Social Psychology, 13,* 405-414.

Howerton, M. W., Bell, B. S., Dodd, K. W., Berrigan, D., Stozenberg-Solomon, R., and Nebeling, L. (2007). School-based nutrition programs produced a moderate increase in fruit and vegetable consumption: Meta and pooling analyses from seven studies. *Journal of Nutrition Education and Behavior, 39,* 186-196.

Knai, C., Pomerlau, J., Lock, K., and McKee, M. (2006). Getting children to eat more fruit and vegetables: A systematic review. *Preventive Medicine, 42,* 85-95.

Perry, C. L., Bishop, D. B., Taylor, G., Murray, D. M., Mays, R. W., Dudovitz, B. S., Smyth, M., and Story, M. (1998). Changing fruit and vegetable consumption among children: The 5-a-Day Power Plus program in St. Paul, Minnesota. *American Journal of Public Health, 88,* 603-609.

Reynolds, K. D., Franklin, F. A., Leviton, L. C., Maloy, J., Harrington, K. T., Yaroch, A. L., Person, S., and Jester, P. (2000). Methods, results, and lessons learned from process evaluation of the High-5 school-based nutrition intervention. *Health Education and Behavior, 27,* 177-186.

Rolls, B. J., Roe, L. S., and Meengs, J. S. (2004). Salad and satiety: Energy density and portion size of a first-course salad affect energy intake at lunch. *Journal of the American Dietetic Association, 104,* 1570-1576.

Rolls, B. J., Rolls, E. T., Rowe, E. A., and Sweeney, K. (1981). Sensory specific satiety in man. *Physiology and Behavior, 27,* 137-142.

Simons-Morton, B. G., Forthofer, R., Huang, I. W., Baranowski, T., Reed, D. B., and Fleishman, R. (1992). Reliability of direct observation of school children's consumption of bag lunches. *Journal of the American Dietetic Association, 92,* 219-221.

Wardle, J., Herrera, M. L., Cooke, L., and Gibson, E. L. (2003). Modifying children's food preferences: The effects of exposure and reward on acceptance of an unfamiliar vegetable. *European Journal of Clinical Nutrition, 57*, 341-348.

In: Fruit and Vegetable Consumption and Health
Editors: Anton Papareschi and Harvey Eppolito

ISBN: 978-1-60741-596-1

Chapter IX

Fruit and Vegetable Consumption among Mid-Age and Older Women in Australia*

Zumin Shi*† *and Julie Byles
Research Centre for Gender, Health and Ageing
The University of Newcastle, Newcastle, Australia

Abstract

Fruits and vegetables are essential components of a healthy diet. However, only limited information is available about the fruit and vegetable intake of older women. This study describes the socio-demographic and health correlates of intake of fruit and vegetables among two large cohorts of Australian women – one group aged 50-55 years and one aged 79-84 years. Almost all women ate some amount of fruit and vegetables each day. In each cohort, around 8-9% of the women ate five or more serves of vegetables each day, and 30% ate four or more serves each day. In the Mid-age cohort, around 60% of the women ate two or more servings of fruit each day, and the corresponding proportion for the older cohort was 70%. Around 7-8% of each cohort could be considered to eat the national recommended intake of two serves of fruit and five serves of vegetables. Eating higher levels of fruit and vegetables was associated with country of birth, education, marital status, and with functional abilities and oral health. Longitudinal analyses describe trends in BMI, health-related quality of life and survival according to women's fruit and vegetable intakes.

---

* A version of this chapter was also published in *Nutrition for the Middle Aged and Elderly*, edited by N. E. Bernhardt, A. M. Kasko published by Nova Science Publishers, Inc. It was submitted for appropriate modifications in an effort to encourage wider dissemination of research.

† Research Fellow, Newcastle Institute of Public Health – Hunter Medical Research Institute, Faculty of Health, The University of Newcastle, phone 49138643, 49138321 or 49138142. fax 49138323. email: julie.byles@newcastle.edu.au

Observational studies have shown that high intake of fruit and vegetables is associated with a lower risk of cancers [1], cardiovascular disease [2], stroke [3], and diabetes [4]. Positive association has also been found between intake of fruit and vegetables and mental and physical function. It is suggested that these effects are mediated through the antioxidant effects of micronutrients in fruits and vegetables such as vitamin C, vitamin E, and carotenoids [5]. Dietary fiber from fruits and vegetables may also add health benefits [4]. However, antioxidant supplement trials on the prevention of cancer and cardiovascular disease show inconsistent or discouraging results, including the Alpha-Tocopherol Beta-Carotene (ATBC) study and the CARET study [6, 7]. It is still debatable whether vitamin supplementation should be used for the prevention of chronic disease [8]. At present, data do not justify the use of antioxidant vitamin supplements for diabetes and CVD risk reduction [9-11]. The beneficial effects of fruits and vegetables can not be explained only by known chemicals, and available studies suggest that the whole diet or food is more important rather than single nutrients. For disease prevention and health promotion we ought to focus on these foods as a whole.

It is recommended by the World Health Organisation that adults should eat 400-500 grams fruits and vegetables everyday [4]. Intervention programs focusing on increasing intakes of fruit and vegetables have been implemented in many countries. For instance Australia has been running a "go for 2 and 5 campaign" to encourage consumption of at least two serves of fruit and five serves of vegetables each day (http://www.gofor2and5.com.au). However, many individuals do not consume enough fruit and vegetables to meet recommended dietary requirements. In Australia, it has been estimated that only around 11% of adults consume the recommended two serves of fruit and five serves of vegetables a day [12] and women living alone are less likely to meet recommendations for vegetable intake [13].

Socioeconomic characteristics are high among the many factors that are associated with fruit and vegetable intake [14]. However, the association between socio-economic factors and intake of fruit and vegetable varies in developed and developing countries. In developed countries, high intake of fruit and vegetable is seen in high socio-economic groups; while the opposite association is found in developing countries. Findings in the USA, Australia and some European countries have shown that individuals with low education, working in blue-collar occupations or with low incomes have less healthy diets that are lower in fruits and vegetables than those with higher education, in professional occupations and with high incomes [15, 16]. In Europe, the difference in the intake of fruit is 24.3g/person/day between men in the highest level of education and those in the lowest level of education; this difference was 33.6g/person/day for women [16]. One study of Australian women shows that individual and social factors only partly mediated socioeconomic variations in fruit and vegetable consumption [17]. Lifestyle factors are also associated with fruit and vegetable intake. Healthy lifestyles like physical activity and non-smoking usually cluster with high intake of fruit and vegetable [18].

A number of studies have examined whether area-level socio-economic characteristics influence diet. Research in the USA, the UK and Finland has shown that people residing in prosperous areas have healthier dietary behaviours and nutrient intakes than those in disadvantaged areas, independent of their individual-level socioeconomic position. However, studies in the Netherlands and Australia did not show any variation between areas differing in their socio-economic characteristics [19]. The density of fruit and vegetable stores in the local neighborhoods was not associated with fruit intakes in Australia women [17].

Age is another socioeconomic factor that is likely to have an impact on fruit and vegetable consumption. Older people are known to be at risk of malnutrition for a variety of reasons, including reduced appetite, eating alone, disability in food preparation, and reduced access to food [20-22]. Older women may be especially vulnerable to poor intakes since they are likely to be widowed and living alone and because they have high rates of disability on activities of daily living.

From the evidence to hand, it is widely accepted that fruits and vegetables are essential components of a healthy diet, and that understanding the determinants of fruit and vegetable consumption is important to promote healthy eating and good health in the population. However, at present, only limited information is available about the fruit and vegetable intake among older people in the community. This study describes the socio-demographic and health correlates of intake of fruit and vegetables among two large cohorts of Australian women – one group aged 50-55 years and one aged 79-84 years.

Method

Women in this study were from the Australian Longitudinal Study on Women's Health (ALSWH). Two cohorts of women were involved: "Mid-age" women aged 45-50 years, and "Older" women aged 70-75 years, at the start of the study in 1996 (Survey 1 - S1). These two cohorts of women were randomly sampled from the Health Insurance Commission (HIC) database, and have each completed four surveys between 1996 and 2005. More details of the study have been published elsewhere [23] and are available from www.alswh.org.au. Characteristics of the women have been compared with each national census since 1996. These comparisons show that, at baseline the women in the study were roughly representative of women of their age in the Australian population with some over-representation of women with tertiary education and under-representation of immigrant women of non-English speaking background [24].

The overall aim of the study is to determine "factors that affect the health of women". The main measures of health are survival and health-related quality of life (QoL). Deaths were ascertained annually from the National Death Index with matching on name, address and date of birth information [25]. All phone calls and correspondence notifying of death or withdrawal from the study were also logged by the study office and compared with the National Death Index notifications to ensure completeness of follow-up for mortality. For survivors, QoL is measured at each survey using the Medical Outcomes Study SF-36 Health Survey (SF-36) [26], a widely used and well validated generic profile measure examines eight dimensions of quality of life including physical, mental and social well-being [27].

Questions about fruit and vegetables were asked at Survey 1 (S1), when women were asked whether they "eat fruit and vegetables most days", and at S4 when women were asked: "How many serves of fruit do you eat each day?" and "How many serves of vegetables do you eat each day?" Response options were; "none", "1 serve", "2-3 serves", "4 serves", "5 serves or more". For this analysis, we defined "higher" intake as two or more serves of fruit, four or more serves of vegetables and six or more serves of fruit or vegetables each day based on the distribution of total intakes. This definition is conservative since the national recommended intake is two serves of fruit and five serves of vegetables (www.nhmrc.gov.au), but is to allow adequate group sizes for analysis.

Other survey items inquire about health circumstances and conditions such as need for help with daily tasks, and use of support services such as meal delivery services. Comorbid diseases were measured at S2-S4 as self-reported doctor-diagnoses including arthritis, diabetes, heart disease, hypertension, stroke, thrombosis, low iron level, osteoporosis, cancer, depression, anxiety, and Alzheimer's/dementia. Other self-reported health conditions (breathing difficulty, chest pain, tiredness, stiff or painful joints, back pain, foot problems, dysuria, nocturia, urinary urgency, incontinence, constipation, poor memory, clumsiness, dizziness) were also reported at each survey as occurring "often", "sometimes", "rarely" or "never" in the past year. A specific item was added at S4 to enable women to rate the condition of their "teeth, mouth or gums", and the five response options were dichotomised as "good" (excellent, very good, good) and" poor" (fair or poor) [28]. Alcohol intake was measured according to quantity (number of standard drinks – 10 grams of alcohol) and frequency (number of days per week). Alcohol intake was classified as Non-Drinkers (no alcohol), Rare drinkers (less than weekly), Low Risk (up to 14 drinks per week), Risky drinkers (15-28 drinks per week), and High Risk (> 28 drinks per week).

Statistical Analyses

Data analysis was performed using SAS 9.1 (SAS Institute Inc, Cary, NC), and STATA 9.2 (Stata Corp, College Station, TX) statistical packages. Initial analyses assessed the effect of fruit and vegetable intake at S1 on survival and withdrawal and loss to follow-up using Cox Proportional Hazards techniques. Frequency tables were used to describe response frequencies for fruit and vegetable intakes at S4. Relative risk (RR) ratios and 95 % confidence intervals (CI) were used to compare the prevalence of other health problems and comorbidities according to fruit and vegetable intake. The association between fruit and vegetable intake and other health conditions and circumstances was assessed using Chi-square tests. The cell contribution to Chi-square was used to examine the effects within different categories where differences were statistically significant with more that 1 degree of freedom. All variables of interest where $P<0.2$ were entered into sets of multivariable polychotomous reqression models. Separate models were used to identify factors associated with intake of fruit, intake of vegetables, and "higher" fruit and vegetable intake (six or more serves of fruit and vegetables per day). In each set, a manual backwards selection process was used to identify variables that could be removed from the model without significantly affecting the significance of the model or goodness of fit. Statistical significance for interpreting these models was set at $P=0.01$.

Longitudinal modeling techniques using SAS Proc Mixed were employed to assess within-individual changes in health related quality of life (based on SF-36) according to fruit and vegetable intake. Change in the log likelihood and Akaike Information criteria [29] were used to compare models.

Results

In 1996, 13716 Mid-age women completed S1 in 1996, and 10903 of these women (72%) completed S4 in 2004. Between Surveys 1 and 4, 204 women died[5], a further 946 women withdrew and 1663 were missing at follow up from the study due to other reasons. Compared to women who stayed in the study, Mid-age women who did not complete the survey were more likely to be separated, divorced or widowed. Of the 12432 Older women who completed S1, 7088 (58%) completed their S4 in 2005; 1838 women died,[6] a further 2101 women withdrew and 1405 were missing at follow up due to other reasons. Women who did not remain in the study at S4 tended to be in poorer health on previous surveys.

At S1, 97.2% of the Older women said they eat fruit and vegetables most days. Survival analyses indicate that Older women who did not eat fruit and vegetables most days were significantly more likely to die between S1 and S4. After adjustment for potential confounding factors (number of comorbidities, education, area, of residence, smoking and BMI),[7] the relative risk of death for women reporting "no" to this item was 1.38(95% CI: 1.03-1.85). Proportional hazards models of withdrawal or other loss to follow-up from the study indicate that this outcome was not associated with fruit and vegetable intake (p=0.204).

Fruit and Vegetable intakes for women who survived and completed Survey 4 are shown in Table 1. Almost all women ate some amount of fruit and vegetables each day. In each cohort, around 8-9% of the women ate five or more serves of vegetables each day, and around 30% could be considered to eat four or more serves each day. In the Mid-age cohort, around 60% of the women ate two or more serves of fruit each day, and the corresponding proportion for the older cohort was around 70%. Approximately 7.9% of the mid-age women and 7.4 % of the older women could be considered to consume adequate amounts of fruit and vegetables combined if the national standard of two serves and fruit and five serves of vegetables was applied. Applying our less stringent definition of six or more serves of fruit and vegetables approximately 29.3% of the mid-age women and 31.5% of the older women could classified as having "higher" fruit and vegetable intake.

Social and personal factors associated with fruit and vegetable intake in the older women in the multivariable models are shown in Table 2. Area of residence classification was not significantly associated with fruit and vegetable consumption but was retained in the model to adjust for sampling strategy. Older women were more likely to consume two or more serves of fruit if they had higher education levels, and if they had eaten out in the past month. Women were less likely to consume four or more serves of vegetables if they were born overseas, were separated, divorced or widowed. Difficulty preparing meals was associated with lower intake of both fruit and vegetables. The probability that a woman would consume

[5] Death recorded prior to 30th June 2004

[6] Death recorded prior to 30th June 2005

[7] High rates of missing data on BMI resulted in reduced sample size for these analyses and so analyses were repeated with and without BMI. There was no impact on the relative risk estimate.

six or more serves of fruit and vegetables a day was positively associated with higher education, eating out in the past month, and "good" condition of teeth, and negatively associated with being born overseas, widowed, and having difficulty preparing meals. There was no association between fruit and vegetable intake and income, needing help with daily tasks, receiving food services, and difficulty getting to shops. These factors were removed during backward regression with no significant impact on model fit. Odds ratios for the final model were not significantly affected by removing these variables (data not shown).

Table 1. Reported fruit and vegetable intake for Mid-age and older cohorts of women (Survey 4)

	Mid-age women 53-58 years N= 10,903	Older women 79-84 years N= 7088
Serves of Vegetables %		
None	0.7	0.8
One	14.9	21.0
Two-Three	53.9	50.4
Four	21.5	19.5
Five or more	8.9	8.4
	Miss=0.5	Miss = 0.7
Serves of Fruit %		
None	5.0	1.4
One	35.2	27.4
Two-Three	50.1	58.4
Four	7.5	9.7
Five or more	2.2	3.1
	Miss=0.3%	Miss=0.6

More and stronger associations were apparent in the mid-age group (see Table 3). A more rural area of residence was associated with higher intakes of vegetables, and higher education levels were associated with higher intakes of fruit and vegetables separately and combined. Country of birth was also associated with intake with those born in Europe being more likely to consume adequate levels of fruit and less likely to consume adequate levels of vegetables. Women born in Asia were less likely to consume adequate levels of vegetables and less likely to consume adequate levels of fruit and vegetables combined. Separated women were less likely to consume fruit, vegetables and fruit and vegetables combined, and widowed women were less likely to consume vegetables and fruit and vegetables combined. Difficulty managing on income was associated with all measures of fruit and vegetable intake. Needing help with daily tasks was not associated with fruit and vegetable intake among women in this age group.

Table 4 shows the association between fruit and vegetable intakes and BMI, physical activity, drinking, and smoking in each cohort. Among both cohorts higher fruit and vegetable consumption was associated with more physical activity, and lower rates of current

Table 2. Sociodemographic and personal variables associated with adequate fruit and vegetable intake among Australian women aged 79-84

Factors in area adjusted multivariable model	Fruit(>=2servings/day)		Vegetable (>=4servings/day)		Fruit and vegetable(>=6servings/day)	
	OR (95%CI)	P	OR (95%CI)	P	OR (95%CI)	P
	N = 6505		N = 6501		N = 6484	
Education						
No formal qualification	1		1		1	
School or intermediate	1.14(1.00-1.30)	0.053	1.11(0.97-1.27)	0.144	1.13(0.98-1.29)	0.087
High school	1.37(1.13-1.65)	0.001	1.16(0.96-1.40)	0.136	1.28(1.06-1.54)	0.009
Trade	0.89(0.66-1.20)	0.442	0.83(0.59-1.17)	0.281	0.89(0.64-1.23)	0.477
Certificate/diploma	1.82(1.45-2.29)	<0.001	1.35(1.10-1.67)	0.004	1.55(1.26-1.90)	<0.0001
University or above	1.87(1.38-2.54)	<0.001	1.11(0.84-1.46)	0.477	1.56(1.19-2.03)	0.001
Missing	1.06(0.80-1.41)	0.681	1.01(0.75-1.36)	0.951	1.19(0.89-1.60)	0.233
Country of birth						
Australian born	1		1		1	
Other ESB (English Speaking Background)	0.92(0.78-1.09)	0.363	0.68(0.57-0.81)	<0.001	0.85(0.72-1.00)	0.054
Europe	1.41(1.10-1.81)	0.007	0.25(0.18-0.36)	<0.001	0.46(0.35-0.61)	<0.001
Asia	2.09(0.99-4.38)	0.052	0.26(0.10-0.66)	0.005	0.29(0.12-0.70)	0.006
Other	1.53(0.68-3.40)	0.301	1.30(0.64-2.66)	0.464	1.77(0.89-3.52)	0.102
Missing	0.89(0.70-1.14)	0.347	0.75(0.57-0.97)	0.032	0.81(0.63-1.05)	0.119
Marital status						
Married/Defacto	1		1		1	
Separated/Divorced	0.89(0.68-1.17)	0.394	0.73(0.55-0.97)	0.033	0.82(0.62-1.08)	0.166
Widowed	0.90(0.80-1.01)	0.064	0.78(0.70-0.88)	<0.001	0.77(0.69-0.86)	<0.001
Never married	0.98(0.69-1.39)	0.913	0.80(0.58-1.12)	0.195	0.79(0.57-1.10)	0.165

Table 2. (Continued)

	Fruit(>=2servings/day)		Vegetable (>=4servings/day)		Fruit and vegetable(>=6servings/day)	
Difficulty Managing on income						
No	1		1		1	
Yes	0.96(0.84-1.09)	0.513	0.84(0.73-0.97)	0.016	0.88(0.76-1.01)	0.065
Difficult in preparing meal						
No difficult	1		1		1	
Some difficult	0.70(0.59-0.84)	<0.001	0.57(0.46-0.70)	<0.001	0.55(0.45-0.68)	<0.001
Unable to do	0.45(0.34-0.60)	<0.001	0.56(0.39-0.80)	0.002	0.38(0.25-0.57)	<0.001
Eating out last month						
No	1		1		1	
Yes	1.35(1.20-1.51)	<0.001	1.15(1.02-1.30)	0.026	1.26(1.12-1.43)	<0.001
Teeth condition						
Bad	1		1		1	
Good	1.18(1.05-1.33)	0.006	1.23(1.09-1.40)	0.001	1.27(1.12-1.43)	<0.001

Model adjusted for area of residence to correct for sampling strategy.

Table 3. Sociodemographic and personal variables associated with adequate fruit and vegetable intake among Australian women aged 53-58 years

Factors in mutlivariable model	Fruit(>=2servings/day) OR (95%CI)	P	Vegetable (>=4servings/day) OR (95%CI)	P	Fruit and vegetable(>=6servings/day) OR (95%CI)	P
	N = 10404		N = 10390		N = 10374	
Area of residence						
Capital/Other metro	1		1		1	
Large Rural	0.92(0.81-1.05)	0.205	1.12(0.98-1.29)	0.096	1.04(0.90-1.19)	0.626
Small rural	0.91(0.81-1.03)	0.154	1.25(1.10-1.42)	0.001	1.14(1.00-1.30)	0.045
Remote/Other remote/rural	0.90(0.82-0.99)	0.031	1.23(1.11-1.36)	<0.001	1.08(0.98-1.20)	0.135
Education						
No formal qualification	1		1		1	
School or intermediate	1.16(1.03-1.31)	0.015	1.29(1.13-1.47)	<0.001	1.33(1.16-1.52)	<0.001
High school	1.23(1.07-1.41)	0.003	1.18(1.01-1.37)	0.036	1.22(1.04-1.43)	0.014
Trade	1.31(1.04-1.65)	0.021	1.28(1.00-1.65)	0.047	1.31(1.02-1.70)	0.037
Certificate/diploma	1.80(1.57-2.07)	<0.001	1.57(1.35-1.82)	<0.001	1.76(1.51-2.06)	<0.001
University or above	1.83(1.58-2.12)	<0.001	1.44(1.24-1.69)	<0.001	1.75(1.49-2.05)	<0.001
Country of birth						
Australian born	1		1		1	
Other (English Speaking)	0.94(0.83-1.05)	0.279	0.82(0.72-0.93)	0.001	0.85(0.75-0.97)	0.014
Europe	1.46(1.22-1.75)	<0.001	0.50(0.40-0.61)	<0.001	0.81(0.67-0.98)	0.03
Asia	0.89(0.67-1.18)	0.408	0.27(0.18-0.40)	<0.001	0.38(0.26-0.56)	<0.001
Other	1.28(0.79-2.07)	0.317	0.36(0.19-0.67)	0.001	0.70(0.41-1.20)	0.196

Table 3. (Continued)

	Fruit(>=2servings/day)		Vegetable (>=4servings/day)		Fruit and vegetable(>=6servings/day)	
Marital status						
Married/Defacto	1		1		1	
Separated/Divorced	0.67(0.55-0.82)	<0.001	0.59(0.47-0.74)	<0.001	0.67(0.53-0.85)	0.001
Widowed	0.91(0.79-1.04)	0.165	0.58(0.50-0.68)	<0.001	0.65(0.55-0.76)	<0.001
Never married	1.15(0.93-1.42)	0.205	0.62(0.49-0.79)	<0.001	0.75(0.59-0.96)	0.02
Difficulty Managing on income						
No	1		1		1	
Yes	0.81(0.75-0.88)	<0.001	0.87(0.79-0.95)	0.002	0.81(0.74-0.89)	<0.001
Need help in daily tasks						
Yes	1		1		1	
No	0.99(0.78-1.25)	0.931	1.07(0.82-1.38)	0.628	1.19(0.90-1.57)	0.217

Table 4. Association between intake of fruit and vegetables and BMI and health behaviours in Australian women at survey 4

		Fruit (servings/day) %				Vegetable (servings/day) %				FV (servings/day) %			
		<=1	2-3	>=4	p	<=1	2-3	>=4	p	<=2	2-5	>=6	p
Old cohort													
BMI	n												
<20	659	**36.0**	**52.3**	11.7		21.2	48.5	30.4		**13.0**	56.4	30.5	
20-25	2,703	28.8	58.9	12.4		19.6	49.9	30.6		9.5	58.8	31.7	
25-30	2,070	26.6	59.4	14.0	<0.001	20.2	51.3	28.5	0.220	8.4	60.6	31.0	0.016
>30	872	28.5	60.5	10.9		23.1	49.4	27.6		11.0	59.6	29.5	
Physical activity													
Sedentary	2864	**35.9**	54.5	**9.6**		**23.7**	51.9	**24.4**		**13.3**	**61.9**	**24.8**	
Low	1677	25.9	60.3	13.8	<0.001	19.2	49.0	31.8	<0.001	7.8	58.4	33.8	<0.001
Moderate	887	24.5	59.6	15.9		16.8	49.0	34.2		**6.2**	56.8	37.0	
High	1052	**21.3**	62.8	15.9		17.2	49.7	33.1		7.7	55.5	36.8	
Smoking													
Non-smoker	4354	28.2	58.6	13.2		19.4	49.9	30.8		9.5	57.9	32.6	
Ex-smoker	1936	29.4	58.5	12.1	<0.001	22.0	50.9	27.1	<0.001	10.3	60.9	28.8	<0.001
Current smoker	379	45.4	48.0	6.6		31.0	48.5	20.4		**17.6**	63.6	**18.9**	
Alcohol drinking													
Low risk	2,471	28.2	59.1	12.8		**18.3**	51.3	30.4		**8.6**	59.4	32.0	
Non-drinkers	2,177	30.7	57.4	11.9		**23.2**	47.8	29.0		**11.7**	58.8	29.5	
Rarely drinks	1,978	28.4	58.5	13.1	0.004	21.2	51.1	27.7	0.007	10.4	58.8	30.8	0.007
Risky	222	**38.3**	50.9	10.8		21.6	50.9	27.5		10.4	63.5	26.1	
High risk	25	**56.0**	36.0	8.0		24.0	56.0	20.0		**24.0**	56.0	20.0	

Table 4. (Continued)

		<=1	2-3	>=4	p	<=1	2-3	>=4	p	<=2	2-5	>=6	**p**
Mid cohort													
BMI													
<20	436	39.0	48.9	**12.2**		**20.4**	50.3	29.3		**13.6**	56.8	29.7	
20-25	3571	39.5	49.8	10.7	<0.001	15.3	52.7	32.1	0.005	9.9	60.0	30.1	0.001
25-30	3298	39.8	50.9	9.2		14.0	51.8	34.2		8.4	60.7	30.9	
>30	2515	**43.5**	47.9	8.6		16.1	52.8	31.1		10.2	62.3	27.5	
Physical activity													
Sedentary	1669	**55.6**	**39.4**	**5.0**		**23.1**	51.8	**25.1**		**16.0**	64.6	**19.4**	
Low	2981	46.1	46.3	7.6	<0.001	15.0	55.1	29.9	<0.001	10.0	64.8	**25.2**	<0.001
Moderate	2312	34.8	54.8	10.4		13.1	52.6	34.3		**7.5**	59.7	32.8	
High	3189	**33.0**	**54.6**	**12.5**		13.3	49.6	**37.1**		**7.9**	**56.1**	**36.1**	
Smoking													
Non-smoker	6424	**37.9**	51.8	10.3		**13.9**	52.0	**34.1**		**8.2**	60.2	**31.6**	
Ex-smoker	2934	39.8	50.3	9.9	<0.001	13.8	53.7	32.6	<0.001	8.4	61.4	30.2	<0.001
Current smoker	1449	**58.5**	**36.6**	**5.0**		**25.5**	50.2	**24.3**		**19.6**	62.4	**18.0**	
Alcohol drinking													
Low risk	5834	41.0	50.6	8.5		**13.1**	54.0	32.9		**8.4**	62.2	29.4	
Non-drinkers	1651	39.7	47.6	**12.8**		**20.1**	47.7	32.3		**12.6**	56.0	31.5	
Rarely drinks	2564	39.7	49.9	10.4	<0.001	**18.6**	51.1	30.3	<0.001	**11.2**	60.6	28.2	<0.001
Risky	614	**49.5**	44.3	6.2		**10.3**	53.6	36.1		7.7	63.4	28.9	
High risk	97	**69.1**	**25.8**	5.2		14.3	42.9	42.9		14.4	56.7	28.9	

Figures in bold indicate significant cell contribution to Chi square.

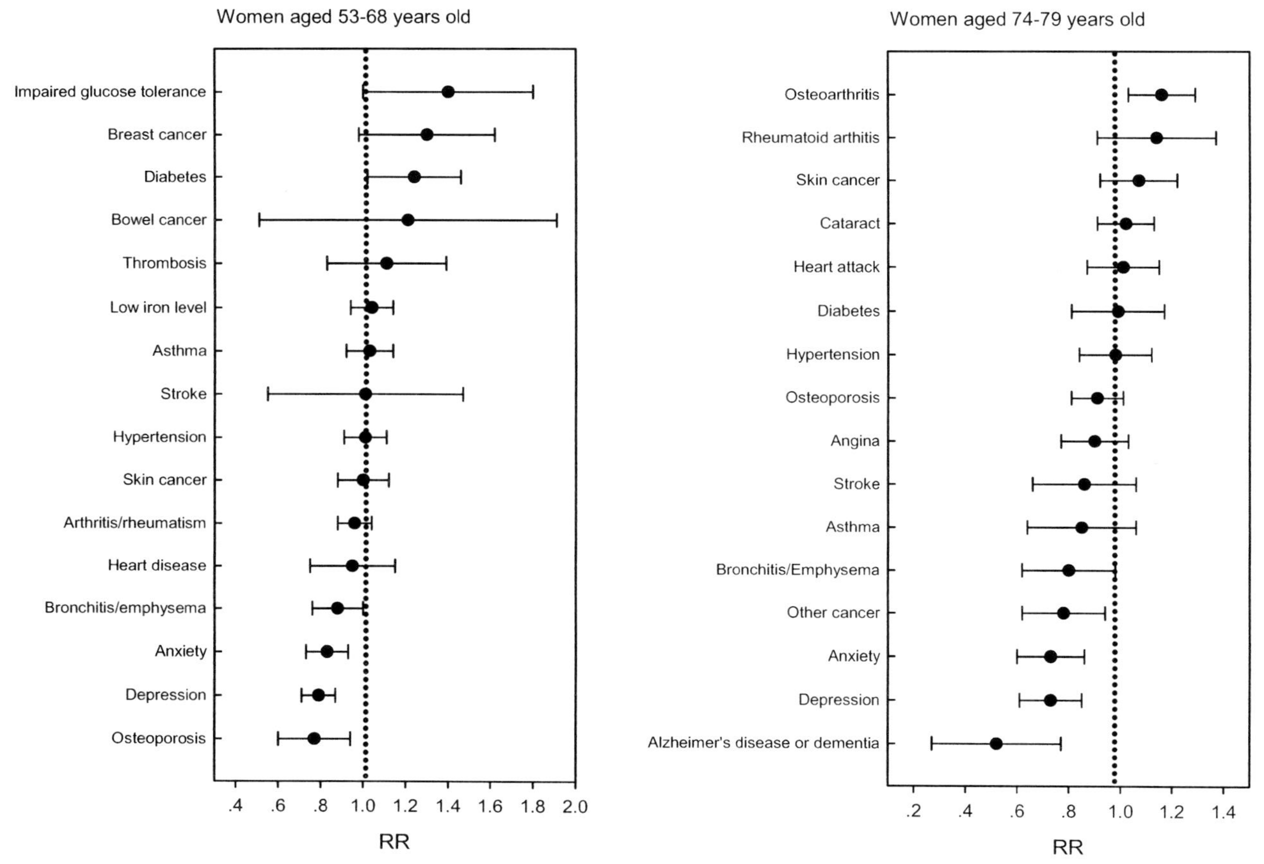

Figure 1a. Univariate Relative Risks for self reporting diagnosed conditions for women reporting six or more serves of fruit and vegetables compared with women reporting less than six serves/day.

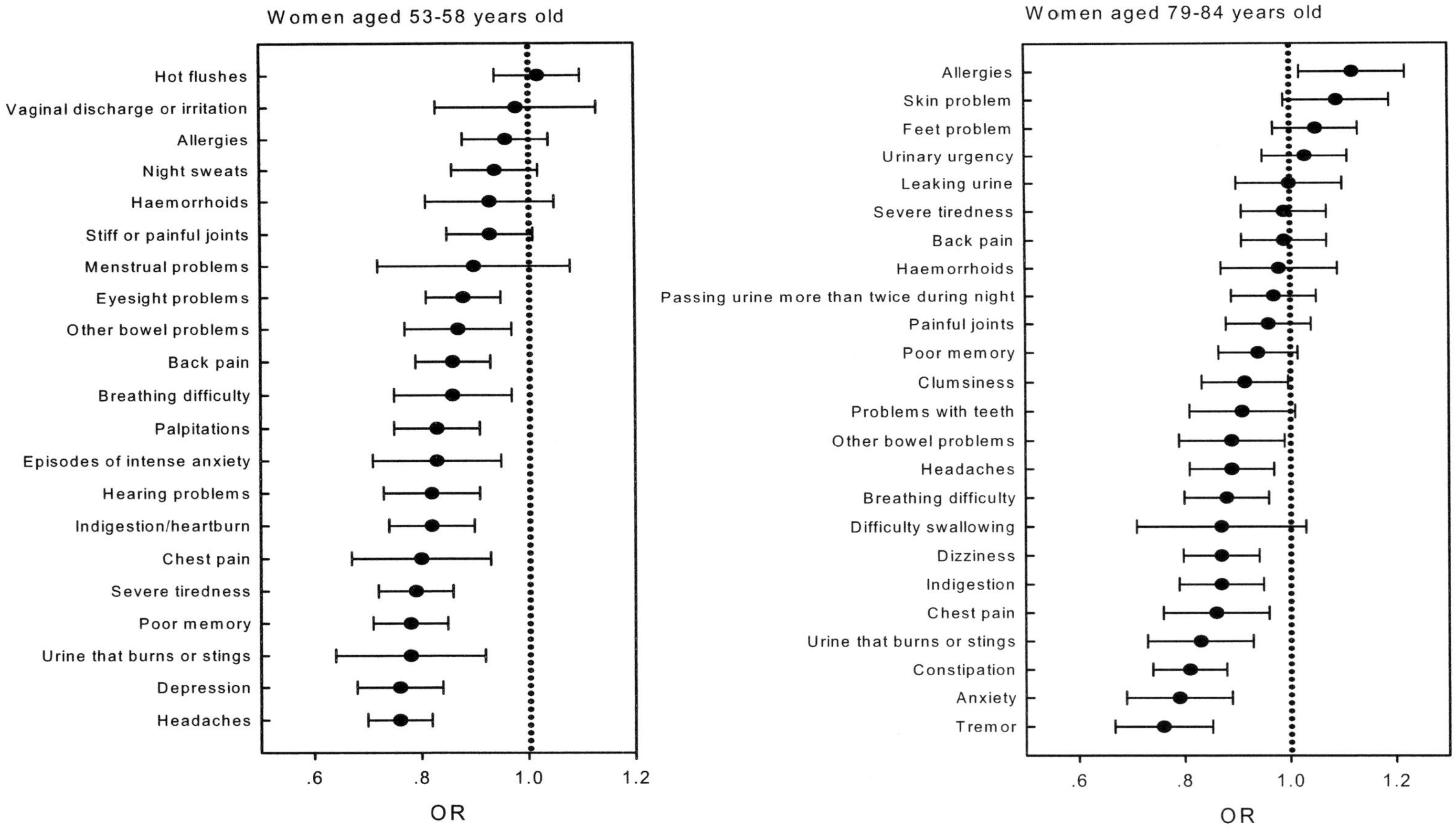

Figure 1b. Univariate Odds Ratios for self reporting diagnosed conditions for women reporting six or more serves of fruit and vegetables compared with women reporting less than six serves/day.

smoking and risky and high risk drinking. While there were statistical associations between fruit and vegetable intakes and weight, the differences were mostly due to only a few cells in the table.

Among the older women, those who were underweight were more likely to consume low amounts of fruit; whereas underweight women in the mid-age group were more likely to consume more fruit and fewer vegetables, and obese women were more likely to consume low levels of fruit.

Figure 1a presents relative risk of comorbid conditions diagnosed during the observation period (S1-S4) for women according to their fruit and vegetable intake, and Figure 1b presents relative risks for reporting other health conditions and symptoms at S4. A number of conditions were less likely to be reported by women who also report higher intakes of fruit and vegetables. However these associations were not strong and upper confidence limits were close to 1.0. Women reporting adequate fruit and vegetable intake were also less likely to report many of the symptoms/complains shown in figure 1b.

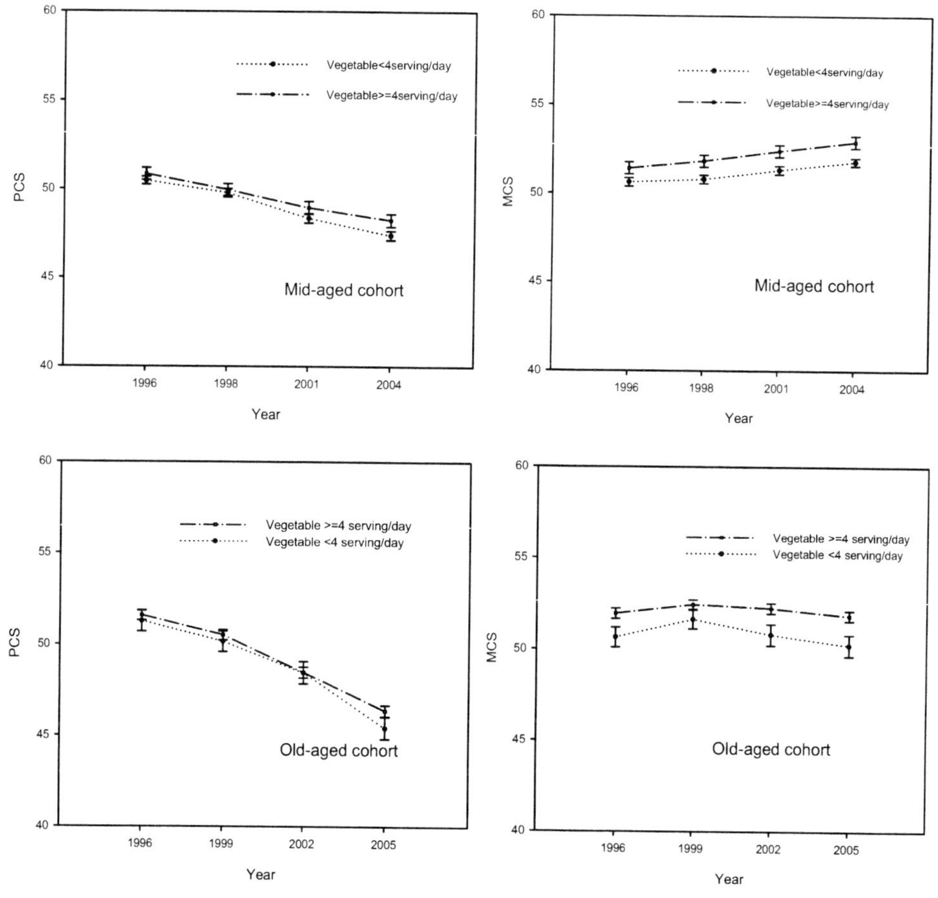

Figure 2. Adjusted (marginal) means and 95% CI for PCS and MCS for women having four or more serves of vegetables and women having less than four serves of vegetables/day. Means are adjusted for age, area, education, marital status, smoking and alcohol drinking status.

Longitudinal analyses described trends in health-related quality of life according to women's vegetable intakes, and the marginal means resulting from these analyses are graphed in Figure 2. In the mid-aged cohort, women who report eating four or more serves of vegetables per day had higher Physical Component Summary scores (PCS) at S4, and higher Mental Health Component Summary scores (MCS) at all Surveys. In the Older cohort these differences were not so clear but the trends were similar. MCS scores were higher at all surveys except S2, and there was a non-significant trend for women consuming four or more vegetables to have higher PCS scores at S4.

Discussion

Fruit and vegetables are deemed to be important components in a healthy diet. The data from this large longitudinal study of two age cohorts of women demonstrate the prevalence of adequate intake among two cohorts of women, and show the strong association between these dietary factors and other health and social circumstances. The longitudinal analyses show the different nine-year trends in health-related quality of life scores for women who do and do not have higher intakes of vegetables the dietary components.

A limitation of this study is that the data can only represent those women who survived and stayed in the study. Older women with poor fruit and vegetable intake at baseline were more likely to die, but were not more likely to withdraw. The association between fruit and vegetable intake and survival is limited by the fact that the women were asked very scant details of their dietary intake at the time of the baseline survey, and the item did not allow much differentiation between different levels of intake.

At S4, the ascertainment of fruit and vegetable intake allowed greater differentiation between women according to different levels of fruit intake and different levels of vegetable intake. The lack of repeated measures of this item over the course of the study prevents an analysis of change in fruit and vegetable consumption and the temporal association between diet and health factors.

It is also a problem that this measure relies on self-report, but this is the method used by most studies of fruit and vegetable intake.

Despite these limitations, the study does provide a large amount of information on women's reported fruit and vegetable intakes and the circumstances surrounding women with inadequate intake and how these women differ from other women of their age group. These contextual factors are important in considering ways to promote higher intakes among mid-age and older women.

Despite national recommendations for two serves of fruit and five serves of vegetables each day (www.nhmrc.gov.au), very few women report intake levels that would meet these standards. There appears to be less of a problem in relation to consumption of fruit than of vegetables. Less than 10% of women in either cohort consumed adequate amounts of vegetables to meet the recommendation. In these data we also do not know what types of vegetables the women consumed and it is possible that one or more of these serves of vegetables could be potatoes which have less micro-nutrient and fibre benefit than many other vegetables. The recommended daily intake does acknowledge that potatoes may make up one serve of vegetables, but if women are consuming more than one serve of potatoes a day then their reported intakes of more beneficial vegetables may be inflated. Australians are known to have high potato consumption and fried potato "chips" are particularly popular among certain cohorts, including mid-age women.

Our categorization of high combined fruit and vegetable intake did not differentiate between proportions of fruits and vegetables in the diet. A large proportion of women would have met this criterion on the basis of high consumption of fruit and low consumption of vegetables, with many women consuming four or more serves of fruit a day. This is not necessarily a desirable behaviour as fruits are higher in sugar and have higher glyceamic index and so may contribute to problems of glucose metabolism (among women with diabetes) and obesity.

The data also indicate that there are clear socioeconomic and personal factors that affect women's consumption of fruit and vegetables. These factors are important to consider if health promotion messages are to be equitable. As it stands, women who are able bodied and who have better levels of education and income may have more ability to consume a healthy diet. The barriers that prevent other women from also protecting their health in this way need to be more carefully understood. It is noteworthy that women who have lower fruit and vegetable consumption are also likely to have other health risk behaviours such as smoking and low levels of physical activity.

While associations between fruit and vegetable intake and the prevalence of chronic conditions were not great, there are more and stronger associations with current symptoms. These immediate benefits may be a stronger selling point for promoting healthy eating than the more distal benefits of disease prevention. Constipation, other bowel problems and urinary problems are particular examples of conditions that are common among mid-age and older women and that may benefit from higher intakes of fruit and vegetables.

Conclusion

The data present a case for further promotion of fruit and vegetable intakes among mid-age and older women who show low intakes of these nutritional components. However in promoting these dietary behaviours some consideration needs to be given to the capacity of women of different socio-economic background to respond to this advice, and to the potential for an unwanted increase in the increase in less beneficial vegetables (such as potatoes) and/or an excess consumption of fruit as an alternative to the vegetable component.

References

[1] Riboli, E. and T. Norat, Epidemiologic evidence of the protective effect of fruit and vegetables on cancer risk. *Am. J. Clin. Nutr.,* 2003. 78(3 Suppl): p. 559S-569S.

[2] Hu, F.B., Plant-based foods and prevention of cardiovascular disease: an overview. Am *J. Clin. Nutr.,* 2003. 78(3 Suppl): p. 544S-551S.

[3] Dauchet, L., P. Amouyel, and J. Dallongeville, Fruit and vegetable consumption and risk of stroke: A meta-analysis of cohort studies. *Neurology*, 2005. 65(8): p. 1193-1197.

[4] WHO/FAO, Diet, nutrition and the prevention of chronic diseases: report of a Joint WHO/FAO Expert Consultation. WHO technical report series 916. 2003, Geneva: World Health Organization. X, 149 s.

[5] Montonen, J., et al., Dietary Antioxidant Intake and Risk of Type 2 Diabetes. *Diabetes Care*, 2004. 27(2): p. 362-366.

[6] Clarke, R. and J. Armitage, Antioxidant vitamins and risk of cardiovascular disease. Review of large-scale randomised trials. *Cardiovasc. Drugs Ther.*, 2002. 16(5): p. 411-5.

[7] Greenwald, P., et al., Clinical trials of vitamin and mineral supplements for cancer prevention. *Am. J. Clin. Nutr.,* 2007. 85(1): p. 314S-317S.

[8] Hemila, H. and E.R. Miller, 3rd, Evidence-based medicine and vitamin E supplementation. *Am. J. Clin. Nutr.,* 2007. 86(1): p. 261-2; author reply 262-4.

[9] Kris-Etherton, P.M., et al., Antioxidant Vitamin Supplements and Cardiovascular Disease. *Circulation*, 2004. 110(5): p. 637-641.

[10] American Diabetes, A., Nutrition Recommendations and Interventions for Diabetes-2006: A position statement of the American Diabetes Association. *Diabetes Care,* 2006. 29(9): p. 2140-2157.

[11] Hasanain, B. and A.D. Mooradian, Antioxidant vitamins and their influence in diabetes mellitus. *Curr. Diab. Rep.*, 2002. 2(5): p. 448-56.

[12] Magarey, A. McKean, S. and Daniels, L. Evaluation of fruit and vegetable intakes of Australian adults: the National Nutrition Survey 1995. *Aust. NZ J. Public Health* 2006 30(1):32-7.

[13] Ball, K., et al., How well do Australian women comply with dietary guidelines? *Public Health Nutr.*, 2004. 7(3): p. 443-52.

[14] Kamphuis, C.B., et al., Environmental determinants of fruit and vegetable consumption among adults: a systematic review. *Br. J. Nutr.*, 2006. 96(4): p. 620-35.

[15] Giskes, K., et al., Socio-economic differences in fruit and vegetable consumption among Australian adolescents and adults. *Public Health Nutr.*, 2002. 5(5): p. 663-9.

[16] Irala-Estevez, J.D., et al., A systematic review of socio-economic differences in food habits in Europe: consumption of fruit and vegetables. *Eur. J. Clin. Nutr.,* 2000. 54(9): p. 706-14.

[17] Ball, K., D. Crawford, and G. Mishra, Socio-economic inequalities in women's fruit and vegetable intakes: a multilevel study of individual, social and environmental mediators. *Public Health Nutr.,* 2006. 9(5): p. 623-30.

[18] Johansson, L., et al., Healthy dietary habits in relation to social determinants and lifestyle factors. *Br. J. Nutr.,* 1999. 81(3): p. 211-20.

[19] Giskes, K., et al., A multilevel study of socio-economic inequalities in food choice behaviour and dietary intake among the Dutch population: the GLOBE study. *Public Health Nutr.*, 2006. 9(1): p. 75-83.

[20] Patterson, A.J., et al., Relationships between nutrition screening checklists and the health and well-being of older Australian women. *Public Health Nutr.,* 2002. 5(1): p. 65-71.

[21] Lipski, P., *The consequences of undernutrition in the elderly*. Nutrition Society Australia, 1995. 19: p. 146-51.

[22] McCormack, P., Undernutrition in the elderly population living at home in the community: a review of the literature. *J. Adv. Nurs.*, 1997. 26(5): p. 856-63.

[23] Brown, W.J., et al., Women's Health Australia: recruitment for a national longitudinal cohort study. *Women Health*, 1998. 28(1): p. 23-40.

[24] Lee, C., et al., Cohort Profile: the Australian Longitudinal Study on Women's Health. *Int. J. Epidemiol.,* 2005. 34(5): p. 987-91.

[25] Powers, J., et al., Effectiveness of the National Death Index for establishing the vital status of older women in the Australian Longitudinal Study on Women's Health. *Aust. NZ J. Public Health*, 2000. 24(5): p. 526-8.

[26] Ware, J.E., Jr. and C.D. Sherbourne, The MOS 36-item short-form health survey (SF-36). I. Conceptual framework and item selection. *Med. Care*, 1992. 30(6): p. 473-83.

[27] Haywood, K.L., A.M. Garratt, and R. Fitzpatrick, Quality of life in older people: a structured review of generic self-assessed health instruments. *Qual. Life Res.*, 2005. 14(7): p. 1651-68.

[28] Benyamini, Y., H. Leventhal, and E.A. Leventhal, Self-rated oral health as an independent predictor of self-rated general health, self-esteem and life satisfaction. *Soc. Sci. Med.*, 2004. 59(5): p. 1109-16.

[29] Akaike, H., A new look at the statistical model identification.IEEE Trans. *Automat. Contr.* AC-19:716-23. Institute of Statistical Mathematics, Minato-ku, Tokyo, Japan, 1974.

In: Fruit and Vegetable Consumption and Health
Editors: Anton Papareschi and Harvey Eppolito
ISBN: 978-1-60741-596-1

Chapter X

A Qualitative Comparison of Fruit and Vegetable Concepts and Knowledge between Preschoolers and Their Primary Care Providers and Childcare Providers*

***Sheila Fleischhacker*[†,1], *Katherine Cason*[‡,2] and *Cheryl Achterberg*[#,3]**

[1] Loyola University Chicago School of Law, Chicago, IL, USA; at the time of the study was a Nutrition Sciences Fellow at The Pennsylvania State University, University Park, Penn State, PA, USA

[2] Department of Food Science and Human Nutrition, Clemson University, Clemson, SC, USA; at the time of the study was a Professor of Food Science at Penn State, PA, USA

[3] Iowa State University; Ames, IA, USA; at the time of the study was a Professor of Nutritional Sciences at Penn State, PA, USA

Abstract

The purpose of this study was to provide nutrition educators with a baseline understanding of how preschoolers' current concepts and knowledge of fruits and vegetables relates with their primary care providers (i.e. parents, grandparents, or foster parents) and childcare providers. The exploratory, theory-based, qualitative study design

---

* A version of this chapter was also published in *Child Nutrition Research Advances*, edited by Laura V. Carter published by Nova Science Publishers, Inc. It was submitted for appropriate modifications in an effort to encourage wider dissemination of research.

† sfleisc@luc.edu;
‡ kcason@clemson.edu;
# docach@iastate.edu

involved interviews with preschoolers (n=24) and their primary care providers (n=22) and childcare providers (n=2). Maps were used to qualitatively compare similarities in responses to questions regarding fruits and vegetables between a preschooler and her primary care provider and childcare provider. The concepts expressed by the preschoolers were shared minimally with their primary care providers and childcare providers. Further work is needed in understanding how to utilize primary care providers and childcare providers and the underlying preschool contextual setting to increase preschoolers' concepts and knowledge of fruits and vegetables.

Keywords: preschoolers, fruits and vegetables, nutrition education.

Introduction

Childcare settings are important—yet under-studied—social environment within which food-related behaviors among preschoolers are developed (Nicklas, et al., 2002). An estimated 12 million, or 61%, of the 19 million U.S. children 5 years of age and younger are in some form of childcare on a regular basis from persons other than their parents (Anne E. Casey Foundation, 2006; Federal Interagency Form on Child and Family Statistics, 2006). The majority of low-income preschoolers receive care at Head Start (U.S. Department of Health and Human Services, 2006). Head Start provides services to an estimated 915,000 at-risk preschoolers and aims to promote early childhood development by helping strengthen the skills of preschoolers, as well as, their primary care providers (i.e. parents and grandparents) (U.S. Department of Health and Human Services, 2006(a); U.S. Department of Health and Human Services, 2006(b)).

Food-related behaviors among children are increasingly problematic. For example, obesity rates have doubled among children and rates tend to be higher among low-income children (Centers for Disease Control, 2006). Close to 80% of children fail to eat the recommended number of servings of fruit and vegetables (Krebs-Smith, et al., 1996; Munoz, et al., 1997; Carlson, et al., 2001). The majority of children also consume too much fat, sugar, and sodium. Low-income children generally have unhealthy eating patterns and are at-risk to maintain these patterns into adulthood.

Both primary care providers and childcare providers can influence preschooler's eating practices by controlling availability and accessibility of foods, meal structure, food modeling, food socialization practices, and food-related parenting styles (Davison and Birch, 2001). While interventions to improve the diets of children, such as promote fruit and vegetable consumption among children in school settings, show potential (French and Stables, 2003), the childcare setting has not been extensively explored. The studies conducted in childcare settings tend to focus on children's nutrient intake or parent participation in nutrition education programs. Parent studies demonstrate that parents tend to have low knowledge on basic nutrition and child-feeding concepts (Hobbie, et al., 2000). In addition, parents are rarely involved in planning meals or participating in other aspects of the nutrition program in childcare centers (Briley, et al., 1999). Entities including the American Dietetic Association and American Academy of Pediatrics provide guidance to assist primary care providers and childcare providers in feeding young children and educating preschoolers on health

(American Dietetic Association, 2004; American Academy of Pediatrics, et al., 2006; American Dietetic Association, 2005). Despite this, few studies examine the relationships between preschoolers and their primary care providers and childcare providers nor the partnership between primary care providers and childcare providers.

Head Start is increasingly focusing on preschoolers' school readiness, in addition to improving the literacy of program primary care providers. Nutrition educators have used books to increase acceptance of a novel vegetable in Head Start preschoolers (Byrne and Nitzke, 2002). Nonetheless, little has been conducted to integrate and evaluate the lessons a child is learning in the classroom with the lessons she is learning at home. Studies focused on parent and teacher agreement on child issues typically demonstrate a lack of agreement between parent and teacher; however, most of these studies focus on behavior, social competence, or educational parameters and not on food and nutrition issues (Cai, et al., 2004; The National Academy of Sciences, 2006; Fagan, 2000).

Designing a study, educational materials, or an intervention for low-income preschoolers can be especially problematic due to the lack of research on this population. According to the Theory for the Ecology of Human Development (Bronfenbrenner, 1979), the Theory of Meaningful Learning (Novak and Gowin, 1984), and the Ecological Model of Predictors of Childhood Overweight (Davison and Birch, 2001), effective dietary interventions must incorporate the targeted audience's context. That is, a thorough investigation of a preschooler's concepts of fruits and vegetables involves understanding a preschooler's settings (i.e. home and childcare), as well as, activities (i.e. eating or helping with food prep and grocery shopping) the preschooler may engage in (Bronfenbrenner, 1979). In addition, the interpersonal relationships a preschooler may have with his primary care provider or childcare provider can provide insight into how that preschooler is developing. For example, when a childcare provider expresses to a preschooler that she does not like bananas, a preschooler can dynamically follow the childcare provider's lead and not eat the banana provided to her at snack. This example illustrates how a childcare provider can serve as a positive or negative role model for a preschooler.

Concepts, according to the Theory of Meaningful Learning (Novak and Gowin, 1984), are a perceived regularity in events or objects designated by some label; are what individuals think with; and are useful in trying to determine an individual's knowledge of a subject. The meaning of any given concept is derived from the interrelationships that concept has with other concepts. One reason, therefore, that early childhood education is important is that it provides a rich base of concepts from which all future learning can proceed. If that base is impoverished, then future learning will be impoverished as well. Thus, a preschooler with few concepts of fruits and vegetables may have a weak foundation for understanding the more complex, but important concepts of fruits and vegetables later in life such as how antioxidants in fruits and vegetables help prevent chronic diseases.

Based on a qualitative study informed by the Theory for the Ecology of Human Development (Bronfenbrenner, 1979) and the Theory of Meaningful Learning (Novak and Gowin, 1984) that compared preschoolers' nutrition concepts to their parents, the study investigator (Achterberg, 1986) concluded that shared meaning on a food and nutrition concept was found to be negotiated between individuals and it is not established between a preschooler and his parents unless there is a defined need, interest or super-ordinate goal to which the parent and preschooler can direct their attention, have an opportunity for social interaction on the subject, and conduct a meaningful discussion about the topic. In the absence of this discussion or exchange, preschoolers created their own meanings for that particular topic. Similarly, preschoolers created their own meanings for particular topics when receiving mixed messages, i.e., from their parents and their childcare providers.

The Theory of Meaningful Learning (Novak and Gowin, 1984) stresses that misconceptions are difficult to change and become increasingly hard to correct as the meanings grow in complexity. Theoretically, nutrition educators need to examine a preschooler's current concepts of fruits and vegetables. Explorations of a preschooler's interaction in his home and childcare center are essential to understanding where to start educating a preschooler and his primary care provider and childcare provider about fruits and vegetables.

The purpose of this exploratory, qualitative study was to provide nutrition educators with a baseline understanding of how preschoolers' current concepts and knowledge of fruits and vegetables relates with their primary care providers and childcare providers.

Methods

Description of Participants and Procedures

An Institutional Review Board at a major research university approved all study protocols. Child assent, parental informed consent, and individual primary care provider and childcare provider consent were obtained. Assent from the preschoolers were obtained once in front of their primary care providers. The preschoolers were also asked for their assent at the beginning of each of their individual interviews. All preschoolers and their primary care providers and childcare providers, with the exception of one primary care provider who could not participate due to her time constraints, agreed to participate. Compensation included child-size water bottles for preschoolers in all six of the center's classrooms. Participating primary care providers and childcare providers received a ten-dollar gift certificate to a local grocery store. Nutrition education for all of the preschoolers, primary care providers, and center staff was provided after data collection.

Study Design and Sample

The primary study center was a Head Start childcare center that had six classrooms. Each classroom was composed of twenty preschoolers and had two childcare providers (one lead teacher and an assistant). This center was located and served a primarily low-income, African American community. The interviewed preschoolers, primary care providers, and childcare providers were recruited from three randomly selected classrooms at the primary study site during January through August, 2002.

The first classroom (n=11 preschoolers; n=10 primary care providers; and n=1 childcare provider) served as a pilot. Based on the pilot findings, revisions to improve the protocol were made including asking the study participants what the word "healthy" means. The subsequent two classrooms (n=24 preschoolers; n=22 primary care providers; and n=2 childcare providers) were used for primary data collection. All of the preschoolers and primary care providers in the primary data collection lived in households below the poverty guidelines and were African American. The preschool sample included twelve boys and twelve girls. The preschoolers' ages were as follows (n=the number of children participating of that age): three-years-old (n=5), four-years-old (n=11), and five-years-old (n=8).

The primary care provider sample included sixteen women and six men. The participants' ages were as follows (n-the number of primary care providers participating of that age): twenty-nine-years-old and younger (n=7), thirty-years-old to forty-nine-years-old (n=13), and fifty-years-old and older (n=2). The participants' martial status was as follows (n=the number of primary care providers participating with that martial status): single (n=9), married/two-parent household (n=9), and divorced (n=4). The number of children in the participants' household was as follows (n=the number of primary care providers participating with that number of children in the household): one child (n-3), two to three children (n=10), and four or more children (n-9).

The two childcare providers' demographics were as follows: one was African American while the other was Caucasian; one was in her upper thirties and the other was older than 50-years-old; both were female; and, both were married with two children.

The interviews were designed according to the study's theoretical framework (Davision and Birch, 2001; Bronfenbrenner, 1979; Novak and Gowin, 1984) and the content of the interviews were used to explore the preschoolers, primary care providers, and childcare providers' knowledge and current concepts of fruits and vegetables. The interviews were also used to explore ways in which primary care providers and childcare providers might partner to influence their preschoolers' fruit and vegetable knowledge and consumption. A prior study demonstrated that semi-structured interviews with preschoolers and their caregivers is a valid means of obtaining information about what the preschooler knows, is learning, and may be exposed to (Achterberg, 1986). Another study showed success with qualitative methods in studying fruit and vegetable procurement and consumption in an inner-city, African American sample (Shankar and Klassen, 2001).

Data Collection

Cards of fruits and vegetables were used throughout the preschoolers, primary care providers, and childcare providers' interviews and included: apple, banana, broccoli, canned peaches, carrot sticks, collard greens, corn, French fries, grapes, green peas, orange, and salad. The fruits and vegetables were selected based on a review of the childcare center's menus and foods thought to be available and commonly consumed in the community. The cards were placed in front of the participants in groups of two or three. Naming the food picture cards was one of the first tasks. The names that a particular preschooler, primary care provider, or childcare provider gave the fruit and vegetable cards were used throughout the participant's interviews.

The audio-taped and transcribed interviews used a structured set of questions with follow-up probes that each study participant was asked to answer. The set included such questions as: what are fruits; which foods here are fruits; where do fruits come from; do you eat fruits; do you eat fruits with other foods; are fruits healthy or not healthy for you; what does healthy mean; and what do fruits do for the body? The caregivers were also asked to discuss nutrition education, grocery shopping, mealtimes, and their interaction with the childcare setting or household. All the interviews of the study participants took place at the center, except for one primary care provider, which took place at the field researcher's home. The order of the questions—i.e., fruit questions first, then vegetable questions—was switched equally among the study participants so as not to bias one section over the other. The preschoolers' interviews were usually about 10 to 30 minutes and took two to six interviews to complete the protocol. The caregivers generally only took one meeting that lasted on average from 90 to 180 minutes.

Data Analysis

The Theory of Meaningful Learning guided the data analysis (Novak and Gowin, 1984). We analyzed the level of shared meaning by comparing an individual preschooler's concepts of fruits and vegetables with their primary care provider and childcare provider's concepts of fruits and vegetables. We also collectively combined and compared the preschoolers, primary care providers, and childcare providers' responses.

The figures or maps used for this study noted the central concept, i.e., fruits or vegetables, in the middle. Then, branching from the central concept were selected questions from the interview protocol. The boxes stemming from the branching selected questions illustrate the study participants' responses to these questions and how they related to their respective preschooler, primary care provider, and childcare provider's responses. Frequency scores were given to each concept to note the number of times this concept was generated amongst the entire sample. Misconceptions were noted with an M. The maps were first developed separately for fruits and then vegetables for each participant. Then, the maps were combined to compare the level of shared meaning amongst a preschooler and her primary care provider and childcare provider. Qualitative comparisons were made based on similarity in responses. Figures or maps selected represent the range in similarities from shared meaning to lack of shared meaning.

Inter-rater reliability was conducted by three independent assessments, including the field researcher. All researchers individually read through each study participant's responses to the study questions. Independently, the researchers noted a study participant's responses to the questions and then constructed and scored a map based on these responses. The researchers also made and compared maps that contained the responses generated by a preschooler and her primary care provider and childcare provider. Agreement on the responses, maps, and concept scores were 89%.

Results

Table 1 demonstrates that the concepts expressed by the primary care providers and childcare providers are similar. On the other hand, this table illustrates that the concepts expressed by the preschoolers were shared minimally with their primary care providers and childcare providers. Common concepts that frequently emerged in the preschoolers, primary care providers, and childcare providers' interviews were dental issues, but these issues did not come out as much in the responses to the fruit and vegetable questions. Children often discussed how candy hurt their teeth and fruit was good for their teeth. Primary care providers voiced the same messages. For example, MBYp explained that healthy is "as in not cavities, not getting any cavities." His four-year-old son had tooth decay and had several teeth pulled during the school year. These dental comments emerged in the fruit discussions, as well as, the primary care providers' discussions on what were their primary health concerns regarding their children. Limited fruit and vegetable availability, as expressed by a preschooler's (MGRp) "no more, no more" description of fruit, was reinforced by her dad (MGRp) who explained that keeping fruits and vegetables, especially fresh fruits, in a full house, on a regular basis was hard.

Similar to the collective sample comparisons, table 2 illustrates that minimal shared meaning was found in the individual preschooler-primary care provider-childcare provider comparisons. One of the few examples of shared meanings is demonstrated in figure 1. That is, figure 1 illustrates how a concept was shared between a preschooler (MGA), primary care provider (MGAp), and childcare provider (MCCP). Figure 2, in contrast, represents the more common finding in this sample: lack of shared meaning. Indeed, figure 2 captures how a primary care provider's (YBEp) response about being allergic to fruit adds insight to her preschooler's (YBE) lack of concepts on fruit.

Table 1. Comparisons between the Preschoolers and their Primary Care Providers and Childcare Providers' Answers for Selected Questions (Number of Times the Concept was Mentioned)

Primary Care Providers (n=22)	Preschoolers (n=24)	Childcare Providers (n=2)
Question: Where do Vegetables Come From?		
Ground, trees, etc. (22)	Store (7)	Ground, plants, etc. (2)
	Out of the woods, etc. (6)	
	Home (5)	
	School (5)	
	Bowl (3)	
	I don't know (3)	
	Stove (3)	
	Meals (2)	
	Barn (1)	
	Cows (1)	
	Food (1)	

Table 1. (Continued)

Question: What do Fruits do for the Body?		
Gives the body vitamins and/or minerals (7)	Makes you strong (5)	Gives it vitamins and/or minerals (1)
Cleans system out (5)	Good for you, help your body (4)	Feed the bones and muscles (1)
Strengthens body (5)	Eat (4)	Helps the body function (1)
Maintain health (4)	Negative things, i.e. make you sick (4)	Provides the body nutrients (1)
Prevent diseases (3)	Make you comfortable (3)	
Fight infections (2)	I don't know (2)	
Keeps you hydrated (2)	Things for particular body parts, i.e. eyes (2)	
Sustains life (2)	Taste (1)	
Keeps weight down (2)	Make you grow (1)	
Makes you feel better, not bloated (1)	Make you happy (1)	
I'm not really sure of fruit (1)		
Makes skin healthy (1)		
Cavities (1)		
Healthier than candy (1)		
Question: What Does Healthy Mean?		
Good for you/helps body (10)	Helps specific body parts such as carrots are good for the eyes (11)	Good for the body (1)
Eating the right things (4)	You eat certain foods (9)	Gives you energy, stamina (1)
Lots of energy, not sluggish (4)	Good (7)	Helps the body function properly (digestive system) (1)
Absence of disease and sickness (4)	Keeps you from getting sick (6)	Provides nutrients (1)
Have vitamins and/or minerals (4)	Bad (5)	Gives you vitamins and/or minerals (1)
Have good eye sight (4)	I don't know (5)	
Fit (4)	They help you (2)	
Provide nutrition/nutrients (2)	Taste (1)	
Sustains life (2)		
Good blood (2)		
Regular, good bowel function (2)		
Doesn't have a lot of sugar (1)		
Strong (1)		
Growing (1)		

Even though limited shared meaning in this sample was found, the qualitative map construction process revealed possible activities that the preschooler, primary care provider, and childcare provider engage in that might help or hinder a preschooler's concepts and knowledge of fruits and vegetables. For instance, in figure 3, YGH expressed several important concepts of fruits and vegetables. Her concepts may have been enhanced by her primary care provider, YGHp, who worked at the childcare center and communicated with the field researcher that she tried to re-enforce lessons taught at the center such as: "She should eat up, 'cause they (vegetables) are good for the heart." Nonetheless, YGHp's vegetable misconceptions, such as: "keep acids out, put acids in," may be a contributing factor to YGH's lack of clarity on whether or not vegetables help or "hurt" the heart.

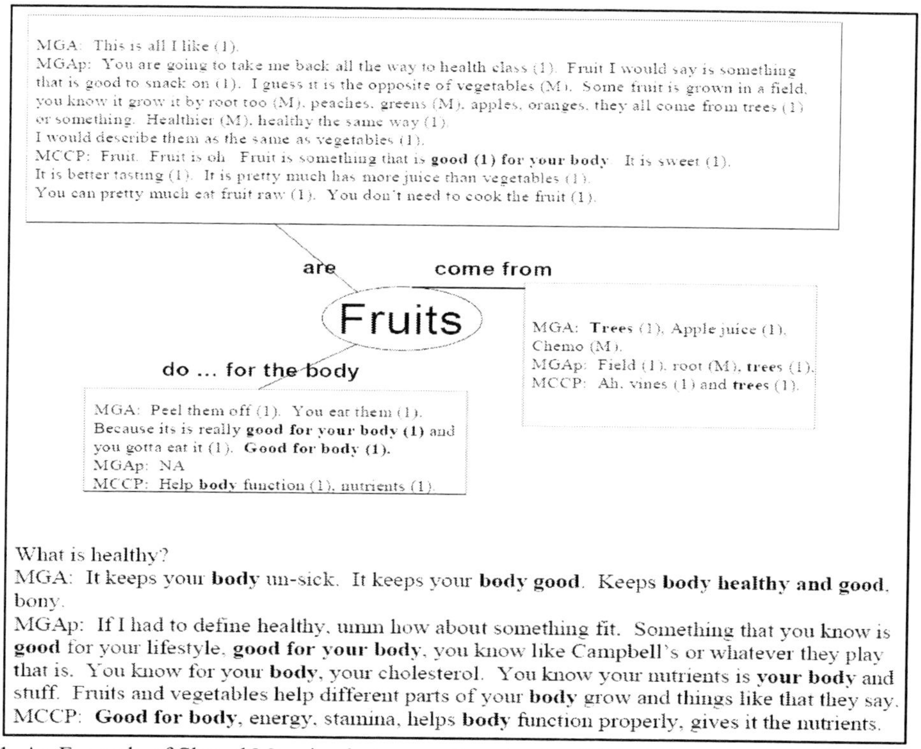

Figures 1. An Example of Shared Meaning between a Preschooler (MGA(5)) and her Primary Care Provider (MGAp) and Childcare Provider (MCCP) on Fruit.

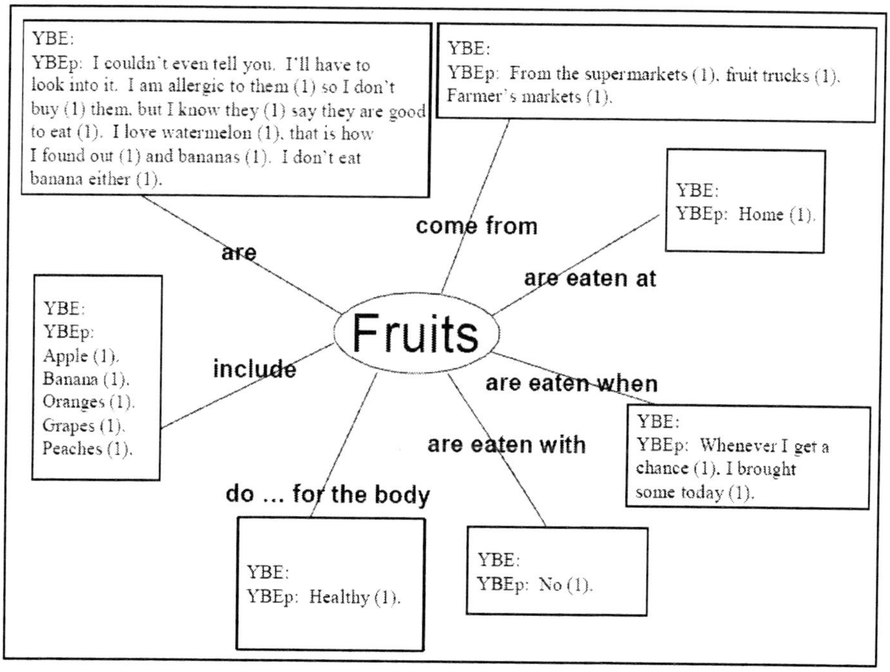

Figure 2. An Example of Lack of Shared Meaning between a Preschooler (YBE(4)) and his Primary Care Provider (YBEp) on Fruit. This map also illustrates how a mother's "allergy" to fruit may have influenced her son's lack of fruit concepts.

Table 2. The Concepts Generated by a Preschooler (n=24) that Matched the Concepts Generated by their Primary Care Provider (n=22) or Childcare Provider (n=2)

Preschooler-Primary Care Provider-Childcare Provider Matching Concept	Frequency of Match
Fruits/vegetables come from trees, ground	6
Vegetables make you strong, gives you muscles	3
Fruits/vegetables are good for the body/you	3
Eat fruit as a dessert	1
Preschooler-Primary Care Provider Matching Concept	
Good for the body/you	4
Vegetables help you grow	2
Fruits/vegetables clean out your system	2
Doesn't eat vegetables at home (child) and don't care for them, didn't eat them (primary care provider)	1
Named broccoli for do you eat vegetables with other foods	1
An apple a day keeps the doctor away	1
Fruits/vegetables are good for teeth	1
Fruits/vegetables help you get healthy, not sick	1
Preschooler-Childcare Provider Matching Concept	
Fruits comes from a tree, bush	2

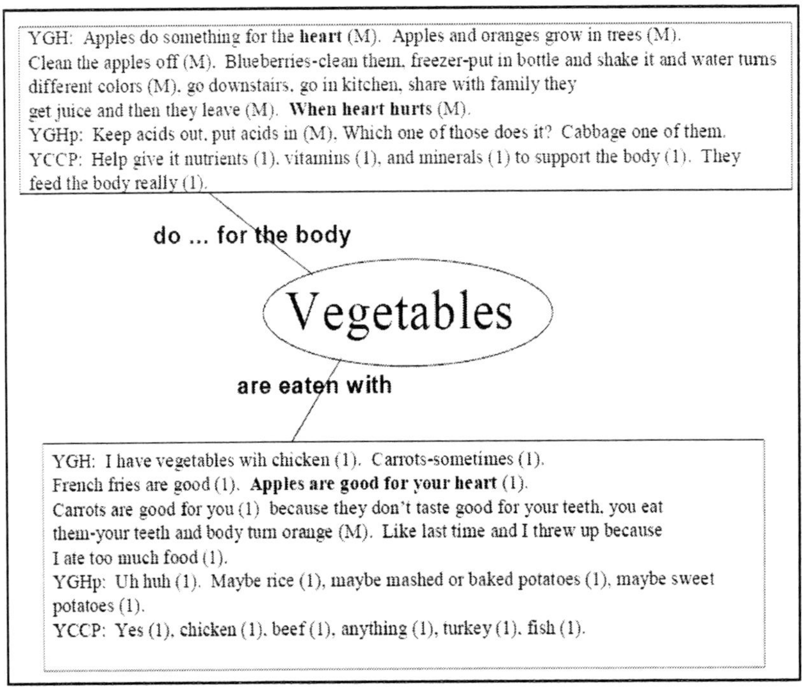

Figure 3. An Example Combined Vegetable Concept Map for a Preschooler (YGH(4)) along with her Primary Care Provider (YGHp) and Childcare Provider (YCCP) Illustrating how Lessons Taught at Head Start such as "Fruits and Vegetables are Good for the Heart" can be Reinforced by the Primary Care Provider (Discussed How She Reminded YGH about the Heart at Dinner) and Childcare Provider (Taught Lesson in Class); But, These Lessons if not Properly Instructed and Reinforced may Contribute to Misconceptions.

Besides shared experiences at the childcare center, a preschooler's concepts and knowledge of fruits and vegetables were enriched in settings where the preschooler engaged in frequent one-on-one time with her primary care provider during a common meal or while grocery shopping. Primary care providers who worked in food service or regularly cooked meals tended to have preschoolers who expressed more accurate and frequent concepts of fruits and vegetables.

The child-feeding practices of the primary care provider and childcare provider frequently emerged during the qualitative interviews and their practices tended to facilitate misconceptions in the preschooler. That is, the primary care providers and childcare providers often mentioned neophobia or the idea of dealing with a "picky eater." Childcare providers explained how they would not serve preschoolers foods "they didn't like" and said: "Oh, they're just picky eaters." Not surprisingly, several preschoolers explained how they would not try any "vegetables" because they did not like a certain vegetable (such as carrots).

One primary care provider (YGKp) discussed how her child's doctor informed her that her child is overweight and is probably going to have diabetes in a couple years. YGKp explained how she would use food as a reward and tried very hard to restrict "the good stuff" (referring to chips, soda pop, and candy) from her daughter with little success. YGK explained that she eats food when she wants to and often until her stomach hurts.

Other types of child-feeding practices or messages that emerged included: "Eat it," "You eat fruit, after you clean your plate," "No juice unless you eat your vegetables, " and "Don't you want a happy plate (clean plate)?" Every primary care provider except one (YGHp) expressed that they portion their preschooler's plate. YGH explained a couple times during her interview how: "If you're hungry, I'll pick some and put it on a plate." The childcare providers did not practice family-style eating, i.e., a child serves her/himself.

The majority of the primary care providers explained that they rarely talk to the childcare providers about food and nutrition issues, but the primary care providers tried to talk to their preschoolers about what they ate at school. One of the childcare providers (MCCP) explained: "We (the primary care providers and I) might talk about food. We might talk about does so and so eat such and such at home because here they don't like it or whatever." The other childcare provider (YCCP) added: "You are not only educating the child, but in a way, you are educating the parents."

Discussion

The results of this exploratory, qualitative study are novel and provide data that may be applied to the development of new nutrition education data collection methods, materials, and programs. Concepts and knowledge of fruits and vegetables in this sample appears to be primarily learned through eating and personal experiences with food.

Limited shared meaning between the preschoolers and their providers implies the participants have limited familiarity with the subject or infrequent meaningful discussion on the subject. Nonetheless, the meanings or lack of meanings preschoolers ascribe to fruits and vegetables appears to have been influenced by their primary care providers and childcare providers' activities (e.g., one-on-one meal time, grocery shopping, or cooking) or child-feeding practices (e.g., don't eat fruit until you have a "happy plate")).

Preschoolers can provide important insights into their food, nutrition, and health experiences (Achterberg, 1986); however, there are challenges to conducting qualitative interviews with preschoolers (Irwin and Johnson, 2005). In this inner-city Head Start childcare center, the linguistic needs and limitations of the participating preschoolers had to be appropriately handled during the interview process and data analysis. Similar studies (Achterberg, 1986; Matheson, et al., 2002) provide a benchmark for our sample as to what is age and cognitively appropriate. Comparatively, our sample demonstrated similar abilities and responses; yet, our sample generated fewer concepts and shared meaning with their primary care providers. In light of the cognitive and educational assessment research on inner-city preschoolers who attend Head Start or not (Karoly, 1998), a finding of limited concepts and knowledge of fruits and vegetables in this sample is logical.

The Theory of Meaningful Learning advocates that educational programs should build on preschooler's past experiences. These preschoolers are aware of fruits and vegetables and can incorporate lessons on foods into their cognitive structure. Therefore, nutrition education data collection methods, materials, and programs based on the preschooler's day-to-day experiences with fruits and vegetables, particularly in the childcare setting, rather than abstract lessons on food groups and food classification, may be more effective in enhancing their concepts and knowledge of fruits and vegetables, as well as, shaping their behavior. Since preschoolers often expressed how they couldn't get fruit until they have a "happy plate," educators may consider working with the preschoolers and their providers on not using fruit as a reward or in a contingent matter (e.g., you must have a "happy plate" in order to eat fruit). Future research could investigate how childcare providers properly naming the fruits and vegetables during mealtime and discussing these foods with the preschooler's impacts their concepts of the served foods and mealtime in general. For example, preschoolers hearing the names of the foods while eating may increase their knowledge of the foods and may even influence their preference for these foods. Early childhood investigators may also consider using mealtime as a more systematic educational venue given that in most childcare settings preschoolers consume at least two meals and a snack—translating into at least one-third of their entire school day.

Misconceptions also play an important role in learning. According to the Theory of Meaningful Learning, if YGHp (as illustrated in figure 3) continues to give her granddaughter mixed messages, such as "keep acids out, put acids in," on fruits and vegetables, then YGHp may actually be interfering with her granddaughter's new learning. Misconceptions are difficult to change. Qualitative research must collect, analysis, and build on the misconceptions communicated by their sample. While this sample did not generate many misconceptions (which is a good thing), the preschoolers and even some providers had difficulty in differentiating between actual fruit and fruit-flavored juices, candies, and snacks. In order to be effective, educators need to know what their participants know and why, such as has misleading marketing messages or product packaging lead their sample to believe fruit-flavored juice is fruit. If educators properly identify the misconceptions and the possible sources of confusion in their sample, then the design of educational messages, materials, and programs will be more effective.

Shared meaning or lack of meaning provides early childhood educators useful data that can be applied to the development of new childcare curriculum and programs. Unfortunately, tables 1-2 demonstrate that the concepts expressed by the preschoolers were shared minimally with their primary care providers and childcare providers. Achterberg (1986) hypothesized that shared meaning about food and nutrition can only occur between parents and preschoolers on topics with which both are familiar. Given that neither the preschooler nor the providers in this sample expressed many concepts about fruits and vegetables, it is not surprising that extensive shared meaning between these individual groups did not take place. Future educational efforts should work on increasing the concepts and knowledge of fruits and vegetables in preschoolers, primary care providers, and childcare providers.

Increasing concepts and knowledge in this sample is a vital step in educating this sample on fruits and vegetables, because Novak and Gowin (1984) explain that concepts tend to stick better when they have multiple meanings attached to them. In other words, providing the preschoolers, primary care providers, and childcare providers with a basic rationale about why to eat fruits and vegetables or a visual explanation of how water, sun, and soil enables fruits and vegetables to grow may facilitate the development of more meaningful messages. These messages also provide a varied venue in which reinforcing groups a.k.a. primary care providers, childcare providers, and other influencing parties (such as the government and health organizations) can build on and branch off of.

Future educational efforts should ensure that primary care providers and childcare providers are trained on appropriate mediums and methods of transferring their knowledge to their preschoolers. In order for shared meaning to be established, Achterberg (1986) suggested that there be an opportunity for that individual to make choices, i.e. to express his or her preference and a social setting where those preferences are observed by, and perhaps discussed with, other family members. This idea of creating opportunities to express preferences or thoughts about fruits and vegetables in this sample may be one medium by which these preschoolers, primary care providers, and childcare providers can increase their concepts of fruits and vegetables. Having the preschoolers express their thoughts about fruits and vegetables to their primary care providers and childcare providers may facilitate more opportunities for the primary care providers and childcare providers to promote meaning, particularly shared meaning, in their preschoolers.

The Theory for the Ecology of Human Development (Bronfenbrenner, 1979) and the Ecological Model of Predictors of Childhood Overweight (Davison and Birch, 2001) emphasize the influence activities can play in a preschooler's development. The primary activities the preschoolers engaged in where they seemed to learn the most about fruits and vegetables was: mealtime, grocery shopping, and cooking. Future work is needed in exploring how activities such as mealtime, grocery shopping, and cooking in either the childcare or home setting may serve as fruitful methods of educating preschoolers. These activities give providers the opportunity to talk and show preschoolers fruits and vegetables. In addition, these activities serve as consistent, familiar, convenient, and fun outlets where fruits and vegetables can be purchased and consumed. For example, health professionals can research the effectiveness of table talk, i.e. lessons a preschooler can learn while eating, such as food identification. Educators should give special attention to the local fruit and vegetable availability when designing curriculum in low-income populations where limited fresh produce is available or affordable.

Books did not emerge as a critical point of learning about fruits and vegetables in this sample; however, given the school readiness focus of Head Start (U.S. Health and Human Services, 2006(a); and U.S. Health and Human Services, 2006(b)), health professionals could potentially develop, implement, and evaluate the use of literacy-based fruit and vegetable lessons, i.e. the use of books. Moreover, further work is needed in understanding how to encourage providers to use role modeling to encourage food acceptance in preschoolers (Hendy and Raudenbush, 2000). Child-feeding practices are instrumental in creating healthy dietary patterns and messages in preschoolers. Our data imply that further work is needed in exploring the child-feeding practices in this sample. Early childhood educators may want to team with child psychologists to develop means of managing preschoolers' behavior without using food as a reward.

Both of the childcare providers expressed how they communicated with the preschoolers and the primary care providers about food. The childcare providers felt as if they were educating not only the preschooler but also the primary care provider. More work is needed in understanding how to connect concise and precise communication efforts between the preschooler, childcare provider, and primary care provider. Educators may consider the use of the center menu or posting lessons learned at mealtime by the classroom's sign-in/out sheet.

This was an exploratory, qualitative study based in one community. As one of the first research studies in this center, the study needed to ensure that its procedures, content, and activities were fun, friendly, and feasible for the participants. The study needed to work on making all methods and interpretations context-sensitive. These steps aided in not only ensuring study collection by enough participants but also set the stage for future projects. We acknowledge the study's limitations: a small sample size and the study focused on only a select sample of fruits and vegetables. The study only used one primary care provider where in some instances multiple caregivers may feed and influence the interviewed preschooler. The sample size of childcare providers (n=2) is particularly small; yet, the size is logical. This sample size provides an understanding of the key childcare providers in the studied preschooler's lives. These exploratory findings do not provide substantial foundation for how concepts and knowledge operate in childcare providers. Nonetheless, the interviews may guide future education efforts and qualitative methodologies on how to connect the preschooler, primary care provider, and childcare provider. Our hope is that future research will address some of these limitations. These findings, in spite of these shortcomings, supplied a foundation for future research and intervening efforts.

Conclusion

The environment a preschooler grows up in has a powerful impact on how that preschooler develops and how that preschooler learns. This impact affects more than just the traditionally targeted and measured educational, behavioral, and social competence parameters. The early years are critical to food-related behaviors and health outcomes. Health professionals are increasingly playing a role in how preschoolers' food-related behaviors are developing in the home and childcare setting.

Based on the results of this exploratory study, we conclude that preschoolers in this inner-city Head Start childcare center have limited concepts and knowledge of fruits and vegetables and have a lack of shared meaning on the subject with their providers. More research is needed in understanding how to increase concepts and knowledge of fruits and vegetables in preschoolers and their providers. In addition, further work is needed in exploring methods and mediums of how primary care providers and childcare providers can individually and collectively transfer concepts and knowledge of fruits and vegetables effectively to their preschoolers.

Acknowledgements

The United States Department of Agriculture Food and Nutrition Services Food Stamp Nutrition Education Program (Fund Number 89EM) and The Children, Families, and Youth Consortium of The Pennsylvania State University provided financial support. Leann Birch, Linda Burton, Tracy Fleischhacker, Terryl Hartman, Linda Kronheim, and Carla Miller were of great help during the research process. Thanks are also due to the children, primary care providers, and Head Start workers who participated in this study.

References

Achterberg C.L. (1986). The Meaning of Food and Nutrition in Families with Young Children: A Study in Social Cognition. Thesis prepared for Cornell University.

American Academy of Pediatrics, American Public Health Association, National Resource Center for Health and Safety in Child Care. Caring for Our Children: National Health and Safety Performance Standards: Guidelines for Out-of-Home Child Care. 2nd ed. Available at: *http://nrc.uchsc.edu/CFOC/PDFVerson/National% 20Health%20and% 20Safety% 20Performance%20Standards.pdf.* Accessed , 2006.

American Dietetic Association. (2004). Position of the American Dietetic Association: Dietary guidelines for healthy children ages 2-11 years. *J. Am. Diet. Assoc.* 104, 660-677.

American Dietetic Association. (2005). Position of the American Dietetic Association: Benchmarks for nutrition programs in child care settings. *J. Am. Diet. Assoc.* 105, 979-986.

Anne E. Casey Foundation. Kids Count 2004 Data Book Online. Available at: *http://www.aeof.org*. Accessed March 7th, 2006.

Briley M.E., Jastrow S., Vickeers J., and Roberts-Gray C. (1999). Dietary intake at child-care centers and away: Are parents and care providers working as partners or at cross purposes? *J. Am. Diet. Assoc.* 99, 950-954.

Briley M.E., Roberts-Gray C., and Simpson D. (1994). Identification of factors that influence the menu of childcare centers: a grounded theory approach. *J. Am. Diet. Assoc.* 94, 276-281.

Bronfenbrenner U. (1979). The Ecology of Human Development: Experiments by Nature and Design. Cambridge, MA: Harvard University Press.

Bruening K.S., Gilbride J.A., Passannnate M.R., and McClowry S. (1999). Dietary intake and health outcomes among young children attending 2 urban day-care centers. *J. Am. Diet. Assoc.* 99, 1529-1535.

Byrne E., and Nitzke S. (2002). Preschool children's acceptance of a novel vegetable following exposure to messages in a storybook. *J. Nutr. Educ. Behav.* 34, 211-214.

Cai X., Kaiser A.P., and Hancock T.B. (2004). Parent and teacher agreement on child behavior checklist items in a sample of preschoolers from low-income and predominantly African American families. *J. Clin. Child. Adolesc. Psychol.* 33, 303-12.

Carlson A., Lino M., Gerrier S., and Basiotis P.P. Report card on the diet quality of children ages 2 to 9. (2001). *Nutrition Insight 25.* Washington, D.C.: U.S. Depart Agriculture Center for Nutrition Policy and Promotion.

Center for Disease Control. America's children: Key national indicators of well-being 2005. Available at: http: //www.childstats.gov/americaschildren/. Accessed March 7th, 2006.

Davison K.K., and Birch L.L. (2001). Childhood overweight: a contextual model and recommendations for future research. *Obes. Rev.* 2, 159-171.

Fagan J. (2000). African American and Puerto Rican American parenting styles, paternal involvement, and head start children's social competence. (2000). Merrill-Palmer Quarterly. 46(4), 592-601.

Federal Interagency Forum on Child and Family Statistics. America's children National Indicators of Well-being 2002. Available at *http://www.childstats.gov/ac2004/ tables/pop8a.asp*. Accessed March 7th , 2006.

French S.A., and Stables G. (2003). Environmental interventions to promote vegetable and fruit consumption among youth in school settings. *Prev. Medicine.* 37, 593-610.

Havas S., Heimendinger J., Reynolds K., Baranowski T., Nicklas T.A., Bishop D., Buller D., Sorensen G., Beresford S.A., Cowan A., and Damron. (1994). 5-A-Day for Better Health: a new research initiative. *J. Am. Diet. Assoc.* 94, 32-36.

Hendy H.M., and Raudenbush B. (2000). Effectiveness of teacher modeling to encourage food acceptance in preschool children. *Appetite.* 34, 61-76.

Hobbie C., Baker S., and Bayerl C. (2000). Parental understanding of basic infant nutrition: Misinformed feeding choices. *J. Pediatr. Health Care.* 14, 26-31.

Irwin L.G., Johnson J. (2005). Interviewing young children: Explicating our practices and dilemmas. *Qualitative Health Res.* 15, 821-831.

Karoly L.A., Greenwood P.W., Everingham S.S., Hoube J., Kilburn R.M., Rydell P., Sanders M., Chiesa J. (1998). *Investing in Our Children.* Santa Monica: Rand.

Krebs-Smith S.M., Cook D.A., Subar A.F., Cleveland L., Friday J., and Kahle L.L.. (1996). Fruit and vegetable intakes of children and adolescents in the United States. *Arch. Pediatr. Adolesc. Med.* 150, 81-86.

Munoz K.A., Krebs-Smith S.M., Ballard-Barbash R., and Cleveland L.E. (1997). Food intakes of U.S. children and adolescents compared with recommendations. *Pediatrics*. 100, 323-329.

Nicklas, T.A., Baranowski T., Baranowski J.C., Cullen K., Rittenberry L., and Olvera N. (2002). Family and child-care provider influences on preschool children's fruit, juice, and vegetable consumption. *Nutr. Rev.* 59(7), 224-235.

Novak J.D., and Gowin D.B. (1984). *Learning How to Learn.* Cambridge: Cambridge University Press.

Shankar S., Klassen A. (2001). Influences on fruit and vegetable procurement and consumption among urban African-American public housing residents, and potential strategies for intervention. Family Economics Nutr. Rev. 13(2), 34-46.

The National Academy of Sciences. Eager to Learn: Educating Our Preschoolers. Available at: *http:///www.nap.edu/openbook/0309068363/html.1.html.* Accessed March 7th, 2006.

U.S. Department of Agriculture and U.S. Depart of Health and Human Services. (2005). Dietary Guidelines for Americans. 4th ed. Home and Garden Bulletin. No. 232.

U.S. Department of Agriculture. Human Nutrition Information Services. (1992). Food Guide Pyramid: a Guide to Daily Choices. Washington, D.C.: Home and Garden Bulletin. No. 252.

U.S. Department of Health and Human Services. Administration on Children, Youth, and Families Information Memorandum. Available at: *http://www.headstartinfo.org/publications/im04/im04_04.htm.* Accessed February 6th, 2006b.

U.S. Department of Health and Human Services. HHS Fact Sheet. Available at: *www.hhs.gov/news.* Accessed February 6th, 2006a.

Index

A

B

C

D

E

I

J

N

O

P

S

T

U

V